Diagnosis in color

Medical Mycology

Gillian Midgley
BSc PhD

Department of Medical Mycology
St John's Institute of Dermatology
St Thomas' Hospital
London, UK

Yvonne M Clayton
BSc PhD

Department of Medical Mycology
St John's Institute of Dermatology
St Thomas' Hospital
London, UK

Professor Roderick J Hay
DM FRCP FRCPath

St John's Institute of Dermat
Guy's Hospital
London, UK

D1350508

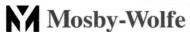 **Mosby-Wolfe**

Chicago • London • Philadelphia
St Louis • Sydney • Tokyo

Related titles published in Mosby–Wolfe's Diagnosis in color series:

The Nail in Clinical Diagnosis 2/e: Beaven & Brooks
ENT Diagnosis 3/e: Bull
Infectious Diseases 3/e: Emond, Rowland & Welsby
Surgical Diagnosis: Greig
Medical Microbiology: Hart & Shears
Breast Diseases: Mansel & Bundred
Skin Signs in Clinical Medicine: Savin, Hunter & Hepburn
Obstetrics and Gynaecology: Symonds & Macpherson

Cardiology: Timmis & Brecker
Pediatrics: Taylor & Raffles
Oro-Facial Diseases 2/e: Tyldesley
Oral Medicine 2/e: Tyldesley
Levene's Dermatology 2/e: White
STD & AIDS 2/e : Wisdom & Hawkins
Physical Signs in General Medicine 2/e: Zatouroff

Publisher: **Rebecca Whitehead**

Development Editor: **Gina Almond**

Project Manager: **Richard Foulsham**

Design: **Greg Smith**

Cover Design: **Lara Last**

Index: **Jill Halliday**

Published in 1997 by Mosby–Wolfe, an imprint of Mosby International (a division of Times Mirror International Publishers Limited).

Printed in Spain by Keslan Servicios Gráficos
Originated by Prospect Litho, UK.
Set in 9.75 point Branding Sans Roman

ISBN 07234 2450 0

For full details of all Mosby International titles, please write to Mosby International, Lynton House, 7–12 Tavistock Square, London WC1H 9LB, England, UK.

Cataloguing in Publication Data
Catalogue records for this book are available from the British Library and the US Library of Congress.

Contents

1 Introduction

Fungi are a diverse group of organisms sufficiently different from other living matter to be considered as a separate kingdom. They are eukaryotic, possessing a nucleus with a nuclear membrane, and have a cell wall composed of polysaccharides, polypeptides and chitin. They show heterotrophic nutrition and live as saprophytes, parasites or commensals on a variety of organic substrates in a wide range of habitats, indicating their global distribution in nature. The kingdom is divided into several phyla of which the *Ascomycota, Basidiomycota* and *Zygomycota* contain animal pathogens. However, the largest number of clinical fungi belong to the Mitosporic fungi, a category which comprises those with no teleomorph, or sexual phase, in the life cycle.

The structure of a fungus may be unicellular – as in the yeasts – or multicellular, where the cells elongate to form filaments or hyphae. These are divided by cross walls known as septa. Some fungi have very few septa and these are described as aseptate. The filaments create a network known as a mycelium which produces the macroscopic form of a mold.

Some fungi exhibit both types of growth and can exist in either a yeast phase or a filamentous phase, depending on temperature. The yeast phase is formed in the host tissue, and at 37°C in culture, while the mold phase is seen in cultures at lower temperatures of 25–28°C. These are known as dimorphic fungi. Other organisms may also produce both yeasts and filaments but the two forms may exist together and their appearance is not necessarily determined by temperature. It is more appropriate to consider these fungi as polymorphic.

The fungal cells may be specialized for certain functions. For example, spores are produced for propagation as a result of mitotic division and also following meiosis if the fungus has a teleomorph or sexual phase in its life cycle. Certain hyphae may be adapted to penetrate the underlying substrate such as plant cells or animal hairs. The basic fungal cell is illustrated in **Figure 1**.

The classification of the fungi is largely determined by morphology. Major divisions are distinguished according to features shown by the teleomorph, or sexual phase in the life cycle, so that the phyla *Basidiomycota, Ascomycota* and *Zygomycota* are characterized by the production of basidiospores, ascospores and zygospores, respectively. Those fungi with no teleomorph are placed in the Mitosporic fungi, formerly known as the *Deuteromycotina*. Further classification is then achieved by comparison of such features as the method of spore formation together with the morphology and arrangement of spores on the hyphae in order to assess the affinities between genera and species. Many fungal species are known by more than one name according to the phase of the life cycle. These will be identified here as the anamorph, or asexual phase, since it is this form which is encountered in the laboratory. Genetic techniques including the sequencing of DNA and RNA are now being employed to indicate a natural classification among this very diverse group of organisms and to provide a solution to the problem of determining the taxonomic status of groups separated by phenotypic characteristics. Details of fungal taxonomy, and full descriptions of the species of pathogens and of their life cycles are beyond the scope of this book and further reading on these aspects is suggested at the end of the book. An explanation of key words used in the description of fungi is given in **Figure 2**.

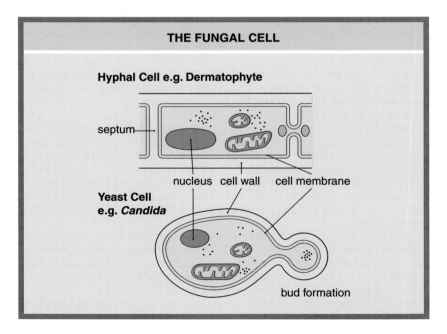

↑ Fig. 1
The basic fungal cell.

Glossary of mycologic terms (part 1)

Aerial hyphae	Hyphae which grow above the colony surface
Anamorph	The asexual state of the life cycle
Anthropophilic	Where the primary host is man
Antler hyphae	Hyphae with swollen tips on dichotomous branches
Arthroconidium (arthrospore)	Conidium formed by fragmentation of the hypha
Ascospore	Sexual spore formed in an ascus
Ascus	A sac-like cell in which ascospores are formed following meiosis
Aseptate	With no cross walls
Basidiospore	Sexual spore formed on a basidium following meiosis
Basidium	A specialized cell which produces basidiospores
Blastoconidium	Conidium formed from an outgrowth of the parent cell
Budding	Production of daughter cells (blastoconidia) by separation of outgrowths of the parent cell
Capsule	A gelatinous covering around a cell
Chlamydospore	A swollen, thick-walled resting cell
Clavate	Club shaped
Columella	A sterile dome-shaped expansion at the top of a sporangiophore
Conidiophore	A specialized hypha which produces conidia
Conidium	An asexual propagule
Dematiaceous	With brown- or black-colored hyphae or spores
Dermatophyte	A member of the *Trichophyton, Microsporum* or *Epidermophyton* genus and which has the ability to attack skin, hair or nail keratin
Dichotomous	Symmetric branching of hyphae
Dimorphic	Having two morphologic forms, dependent on temperature
Diploid	Containing a double set of chromosomes
Dysgonic	A slow-growing variant

↑ **Fig. 2**
Glossary.

Glossary of mycologic terms (part 2)

Ectothrix	Dermatophytic *in vivo* hair invasion where most of the fungus is in the form of a sheath of spores outside the hair
Endospore	A spore formed inside a cell by cleavage of the contents
Endothrix	Dermatophytic *in vivo* hair invasion where the spores are formed inside the hair
Fusiform	Tapering at both ends and swollen at the middle, spindle shaped
Geophilic	Where the natural habitat is in the soil
Glabrous	Smooth or waxy surface without aerial mycelium
Haploid	Containing a single set of chromosomes
Hypha	A filament
Intercalary	Occurring within the length of a hypha
Macroconidium	The larger of two types of conidium formed in a single species
Meiosis	Division of diploid nucleus to form two haploid nuclei
Microconidium	The smaller of two types of conidium formed in a single species
Mitosis	Division of diploid nucleus to form two diploid nuclei
Mold	A filamentous fungus
Muriform	Showing both vertical and horizontal divisions
Mycelium	A mass of hyphae
Mycetoma	A solid mass composed of fungal elements in tissue
Pectinate hyphae	Hyphae which have comb-like projections
Phialide	A specialized cell which produces successive conidia
Pseudohypha	A filament formed by the elongation of yeast cells
Pyriform	Pear shaped
Rhizoid	A root-like filament

↑ **Fig. 2**
Glossary (cont).

Glossary of mycologic terms (part 3)

Scutula	Cup-like crusts containing profuse hyphae, formed on the skin in favus (*Trichophyton schoenleinii* infection)
Septum	A cross wall
Spherule	A spherical cell containing endospores
Sporangiophore	A specialized hypha which produces a sporangium
Sporangium	A structure in which asexual spores are formed by cleavage of the contents
Spore	A general term for a reproductive propagule
Teleomorph	The sexual phase of the life cycle
Vesicle	A swollen tip of a conidiophore or sporangiophore
Yeast	A fungus which is predominantly unicellular and characteristically divides by budding
Zoophilic	Where the primary host is an animal
Zygospore	A thick-walled resting spore. Formed by the teleomorph of *Zygomycetes* after hyphal fusion and in which meiosis occurs

↑ **Fig. 2**
Glossary (cont).

There are several ways in which fungi cause disease in man. These include invasion of tissues by the pathogen and the elicitation of allergic responses in the host. Diseases which follow invasion are known as superficial, subcutaneous and systemic mycoses; entry of the fungus can be
- directly onto the skin,
- by implantation via a superficial injury,
- by inhalation,
- from a previous deep focus of infection in the body leading to internal dissemination.

These are exogenous infections. Examples are dermatophytosis, the subcutaneous mycoses and aspergillosis. Commensal fungi such as *Malassezia* species on the skin, or *Candida* species in the alimentary tract, can take on a pathogenic role when conditions are altered in the host, allowing the organisms to multiply and invade the tissues, so causing the development of endogenous infections.

Immunologic reactions due to the presence of these fungi may contribute to the pathology of infections either at the site of the invasion, as in the formation of granulomas, or at a distance by causing skin conditions such as erythema nodosum, urticaria or vesicular eczema (pompholyx).

Another type of infection is the allergic response elicited by fungal antigens which generally follows inhalation of the spores. It has been estimated that between 4% and 15% of respiratory allergic diseases such as asthma may be caused by fungi. A summary of the mycoses found in man is given in **Figure 3**.

The mycoses

Superficial mycoses
Dermatophytosis, tinea
Superficial candidosis
Malassezia infections
Scytalidium infections
Onychomycosis
White piedra
Black piedra
Tinea nigra
Otomycosis
Mycotic keratitis

Subcutaneous mycoses
Eumycetoma
Actinomycetoma
Sporotrichosis
Chromoblastomycosis
Phaeohyphomycosis
Lobomycosis
Subcutaneous zygomycosis

Systemic mycoses
Endemic respiratory mycoses
Histoplasmosis
Coccidioidomycosis
Blastomycosis
Paracoccidioidomycosis
Penicillium marneffei
infection
Opportunistic mycoses
Candidosis
Aspergillosis
Cryptococcosis
Zygomycosis
Rare infections due to
Fusarium species,
Trichosporon species,
etc.

↑ **Fig. 3**
The mycoses.

2 | **Pathogenesis**

The process of infection of the host depends on a number of factors. Initially, there is the survival of infective spores in the environment. For example, dermatophyte arthroconidia have been shown to survive for over two years in shed skin scales. The subsequent adhesion of fungal cells to the skin or mucosal surface is necessary; this relies on a time-dependent physicochemical bond between a fungal cell wall receptor and keratinocytes or mucosal cells. Skin surface factors such as pH and carbon dioxide tension are also relevant. During the onset of subcutaneous infections the pathogens are introduced directly to the tissues by implantation during injury.

In skin disease certain fungi are able to penetrate keratinized cells by producing enzymes such as keratinases. *Trichophyton mentagrophytes*, for example, has at least two enzyme isotypes. However, this property is not shared by all skin pathogens, for some fungi which cause nail disease appear to be able to invade the nail plate only if there is a pre-existing abnormality such as peripheral vascular disease. *Candida albicans* elaborates a proteinase which is important for determining virulence, since strains which do not produce this enzyme have been shown to be less successful as pathogens in experimental infections. *Malassezia* species produce lipases which may aid the digestion of fats in sebum and provide nutrients for their growth and multiplication.

Changes in host defenses, even minor ones, are important for allowing organisms to invade the skin, respiratory tract or mucous membranes. A number of these are given in **Figure 4**.

The reasons for increased incidence of infection in the presence of certain predisposing factors are varied and include:
- the use of antibiotics, reducing the local bacteria flora that compete for adherence sites;
- in diabetes mellitus, an increase in levels of available sugars in tissues and a reduction of phagocyte efficiency.

The existence of a predisposing factor in the host will not necessarily lead to an increased frequency of infection as this also depends on exposure to the infecting organism. In AIDS, for instance, oropharyngeal candidosis is very common as the yeast *Candida* is a normal oral commensal. Dermatophytosis, on the other hand, does not have an increased incidence in the AIDS population presumably because the frequency of exposure to dermatophytes is no higher in this group. However, the clinical manifestations of dermatophytosis in AIDS patients will often differ from those seen in other subjects.

The survival of pathogenic fungi in the host depends on a number of different properties possessed by the various fungi which allow the growth of the organisms and which protect them against immune destruction. These range from the ability to grow at physiologic temperatures, and cell wall thickening to the production of immunomodulatory antigens and the deposition of melanin either in the cell wall or extracellularly. There are different forms of immunomodulation associated with pathogenic fungi. Examples include:

- *Cryptococcus neoformans*, which is surrounded by a capsule preventing adequate phagocytic killing;
- *Candida albicans* and *Trichophyton rubrum*, which both produce a cell wall mannan polysaccharide residue that reduces T-lymphocyte blastogenesis;
- *Cladosporium carrionii*, which forms a cell wall melanin protecting against oxidative neutrophil killing.

Factors associated with fungal infection

Factor	Infection
Age – infancy, old age	Candidosis
Pregnancy	Candidosis
Epithelial abnormalities	Candidosis, dermatophytosis
Endocrine disease	Candidosis, dermatophytosis, pityriasis versicolor, zygomycosis
Antibiotic therapy	Candidosis, aspergillosis
Iron deficiency	Candidosis
Zinc deficiency	Candidosis
Immunosuppression (drugs, congenital, malignancies) affecting:	
Neutrophils	Candidosis, aspergillosis, zygomycosis
T-lymphocytes	Most, except aspergillosis, zygomycosis

↑ **Fig. 4**
Factors associated with fungal infection.

3 Laboratory Diagnosis

The laboratory methods used in the diagnosis of fungal infections involve the detection of the organism in the tissues, isolation of the pathogen in culture and recognition of specific responses in the host using immunologic techniques or by histopathology.

3.1 Collection of specimens

In the superficial mycoses, evidence of fungal infection is obtained by direct microscopy of the keratin. Material from skin lesions is removed by scraping the site with a solid blunt scalpel so that the scales are collected onto a glass slide for immediate processing (**Fig. 5**), or into a folded paper packet if the specimen is to be mailed. Experience determines the most suitable material, but with a spreading lesion the active periphery is selected as this is most likely to contain viable fungal elements. If vesicles are present, the roof will often reveal abundant hyphae; with folliculitis, hyphae may be seen around the root of hairs from the limbs or face when they may be scanty elsewhere.

→ Fig. 5 Collection of skin material for diagnosis.

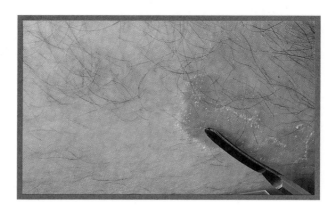

Hairs from the scalp or beard area are removed with a pair of flat-ended forceps. Infected hairs slip out easily from the follicles. However, the best material from the scalp frequently will be scrapings, taken with a blunt scalpel, in which the infected hair stumps are embedded (**Fig. 6**). Brush samples using commercially available circular massage brushes can be used to culture material from the scalp. After being passed through the hair the brush is pressed into a Petri dish containing medium. Infected children will produce colonies from many points of the brush (**Figs 7&8**). This is a useful method to survey siblings and other contacts of infected children and also suspected household pets. Inflammatory painful lesions, such as kerion on a sensitive child, can be difficult to sample; a moistened swab rubbed over the infected area may be the only way to collect a specimen. Positive cultures can be obtained in this way but a negative result would not exclude an infection.

Nails are usually thickened when they are infected and clippers are essential to cut a sample through the full thickness. Any subungual debris should also be collected. As nails generally are invaded from the lateral and distal margins, the youngest and most viable elements will be in the proximal portion which is difficult to sample. Hence cultures of infected nails have a lower recovery rate when compared with skin. The clinical condition of superficial white onychomycosis can be sampled by using a scalpel to remove some of the affected area on the top of the nail. This material is usually heavily invaded with fungal hyphae.

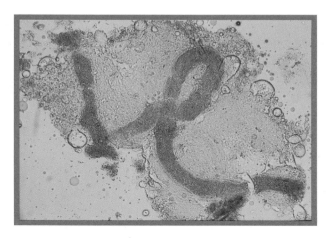

← **Fig. 6**
Infected hair in a scalp scale.

Provided that the material is kept dry, specimens of skin, hair and nail wrapped in paper packets will remain suitable for analysis for several months.

Samples are taken from mucosae with moistened cotton wool swabs which are analysed immediately or placed in transport medium. With the deeper infections sputum, exudates, body fluids, biopsies, etc. are collected in sterile containers and processed as quickly as possible.

**→ Fig. 7
Preparation
of a brush
culture.**

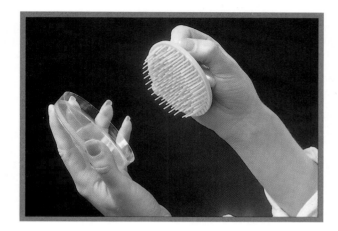

**→ Fig. 8
Culture of a
scalp brush
sample
showing
colonies
produced
from every
point of the
brush.**

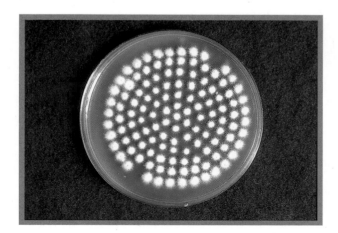

3.2 Observation of fungi in the tissues

Samples of keratin are placed in 10–30% potassium hydroxide (KOH) solution and examined directly unstained. It is essential to allow the material to soften adequately so that a thin layer of cells is formed. Gentle heat may be necessary to hasten softening of the keratin, particularly with nails. Fungal elements can be visualized by controlling the amount of light passing through the specimen and by altering the focus as the slide is scanned. Dermatophyte hyphae are septate and regular in width and they may divide into arthroconidia (**Fig. 9**). If hairs are infected, the size and arrangement of the spores, together with the ability to fluoresce under a Wood's light, will help toward the identification of the dermatophyte species involved (see Figs 49–51&53).

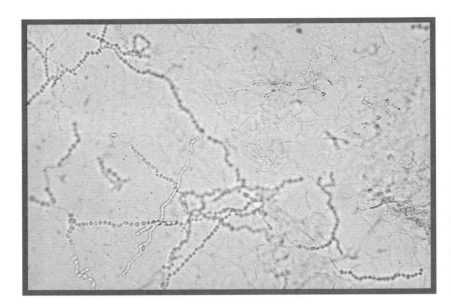

↑ **Fig. 9**
KOH preparation of skin infected with a dermatophyte. The hyphae are regular in width, have septa and may branch.

Other fungi can often be suspected by their appearance in a direct preparation and distinguished from a dermatophyte. Those features will be indicated in the illustrations given in the relevant chapters. The use of Parker's stain (equal parts 30% KOH and Parker's permanent blue/black ink) is particularly helpful in demonstrating the organism in scales from pityriasis versicolor, as the fungus, *Malassezia furfur,* takes up the blue color immediately. It is also of use to indicate some nondermatophyte pathogens in nails. In contrast, the dermatophytes will take up the color only after several hours in the stain.

Before examination, sputum should be digested with sodium hydroxide or *N*-acetylcysteine and dithiothreitol.

The appearance of many fungi in wet pathologic specimens, particularly body fluids, can be enhanced by using calcofluor white but a fluorescence facility must be available on the microscope for this technique.

Smears from mucosae may also be examined unstained, or they may be heat-fixed on the slide and stained by the Gram or periodic acid–Schiff (PAS) method. Pus, exudates and body fluids may be spun down and the deposit examined for the presence of yeasts or filaments, etc. either unstained or after staining by Gram, PAS, Gomori methenamine–silver (GMS), Giemsa or mucicarmine according to the disease suspected. For cryptococcosis, and when any cerebrospinal fluid (CSF) material is being examined, a background stain such as nigrosin or India ink preparation should be included. Sections from biopsy specimens should be stained using the above stains as appropriate.

3. 3 Culture methods

A simple glucose–peptone agar based on Sabouraud's formula is suitable for the culture of most pathogenic fungi. A 4% malt extract agar is also favored by many mycologists (**Fig. 10**). The cultures illustrated here have all been cultured on the glucose–peptone formula.

Sabouraud dextrose agar is available from several commercial firms. As the morphology of fungal isolates may vary according to the particular source of the medium, it is advisable to obtain repeat orders from a single supplier in order to minimize the variation in cultural conditions.

Petri dishes are satisfactory for the culture of fungi and allow for the development of the morphologic features of the colonies which are used in identification. However, it is essential to use screw-capped bottles and the appropriate containment level when handling both material and cultures from respiratory infections, such as histoplasmosis, as these represent a laboratory hazard. Also, for these diseases, cultures may be prepared on a richer medium such as brain–heart infusion (BHI) agar and they should be incubated at two temperatures, 26°C and 37°C, to demonstrate the dimorphic nature of the fungus.

Hairs, skin scales and small fragments of nail are placed on the agar and pressed onto the surface to give a good contact with the medium. Biopsy material should be ground or cut into small pieces. For the culture of blood, vented culture bottles with diphasic media are recommended, as is the lysis–centrifugation method.

The optimum temperature for recovery of dermatophytes is from 26°C to 30°C but *Candida* species, *Aspergillus, Zygomycetes* etc. can be incubated at 37°C. Incubation times vary according to the species. The dermatophytes will take from 7 to14 days to develop but other fungi grow more rapidly, and species such as *Aspergillus* or *Scytalidium*, as well as the yeasts, can be identified within a week. In contrast, cultures of specimens from the subcutaneous and systemic infections should be incubated for periods of 4–12 weeks according to the disease suspected. With incubation times of this length it is necessary to prevent dehydration of the medium so the plates should be poured to give a thick layer of the medium using 25–30ml in a standard 9cm diameter Petri dish. Steps may need to be taken to maintain a humid atmosphere in the incubator, either by adding a water reservoir or by enclosing the Petri dishes in boxes.

Isolation media

Glucose–peptone agar		**Malt extract agar**	
Glucose	20g	Malt extract	40g
Mycologic peptone	10g		
Agar	15g	Agar	15g
Distilled H$_2$O to	1 liter	Distilled H$_2$O to	1 liter

To reduce contamination on primary isolation, the following antibiotics are dissolved in 5ml acetone and added to the above media per liter before autoclaving:

Chloramphenicol	0.05g
Cycloheximide	0.4g

Cycloheximide inhibits the growth of fungal contaminants and provides a selective medium for dermatophytes. It should not be used in cultures for yeasts or opportunists such as *Scopulariopsis, Scytalidium, Aspergillus,* etc.

↑ **Fig. 10**
Isolation media.

Identification of fungi

Fungi are identified by their morphologic features and, to a lesser degree, by their physiologic properties. Macroscopic features such as the texture of the colony, the surface color and the production of pigment seen on the reverse side of the Petri dish can be diagnostic.

To examine a fungus under the microscope, a portion of the culture is teased out in a drop of lactophenol cotton blue on a microscope slide. Some fungi can be examined by a Scotch tape strip where a piece of the tape is pressed against the surface of the colony and then placed on a drop of stain on a slide and viewed directly. This reveals the arrangement of the spores as they are *in situ*. A slide culture will give a permanent preparation of this feature. It is prepared by inoculating each side of a block of agar on a slide and applying a cover slip. After incubation in a moist chamber, when sufficient growth has developed, the agar block is discarded and stained preparations made of the ring of growth on the slide and cover slip (**Fig. 11**).

The identification of yeasts is described on page 68–70.

Serology

Serologic tests are of no value for the diagnosis of superficial mycoses, but various methods for the detection of either antibody responses or of circulating antigen are used to aid in the diagnosis and monitor the progress of the deeper fungal infections. These will be indicated where appropriate.

**→ Fig. 11
Slide culture.**

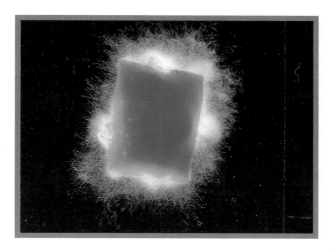

4 | Superficial Mycoses

The superfical mycoses are the most frequently occurring human fungal infections. They include dermatophytosis, superficial candidosis, *Malassezia* and *Scytalidium* infections as well as rarer conditions such as tinea nigra and black and white piedra. Superficial infections rarely extend to deep tissue except in candidosis, although even here most infections arising on the skin or oral mucosa do not invade the host any further.

4.1 Dermatophytosis

The dermatophytes are a group of closely related fungi which have the ability to invade the stratum corneum of the epidermis and keratinized tissues derived from it such as hair or nail. They are related to organisms in the soil which are active in the breakdown of keratinous material. They comprise three anamorphic genera, *Trichophyton, Epidermophyton* and *Microsporum*. The infections caused can be divided into those which are spread from man to man (anthropophilic), animal to man (zoophilic) or soil to man (geophilic) (**Fig. 12**). The initial infection follows contact with an infected desquamated scale or hair and the process of skin invasion is initiated by adherence of the fungal elements to the stratum corneum. Subsequently, these elements germinate and start to invade the keratinocytes. Diagnosis is confirmed by the recognition of septate hyphae with or without arthroconidia in skin scales examined after treatment with potassium hydroxide (KOH) (see Fig. 9).

Pathology
Most dermatophyte infections are confined to the stratum corneum or its appendages. In the skin the infection seldom passes the granular layer unless there is hair follicle invasion, when fungal fragments are surrounded by phagocytes or giant cells in the dermis in the vicinity of a destroyed follicle. In many infections the main feature is a lymphohistiocytic infiltrate around the upper dermal blood vessels, the fungus in the upper layers of the epidermis being visible only with special stains such as periodic acid–Schiff (PAS). In the early phase of more inflammatory lesions there is a dense neutrophil accumulation around hair follicles.

Epidemiology

Dermatophyte infections occur throughout the life span in both the sexes. However, tinea capitis is usually confined to children, and is rarely seen in adults. Tinea pedis is uncommon under the age of 10.

Animal or zoophilic infections are usually sporadic and restricted to the areas where the host animal is found. *Microsporum canis,* the cat and dog ringworm, is the commonest of the zoophilic infections worldwide and spread occurs directly from an infected animal and, possibly, from contaminated furniture, floors and carpets in the home environment.

Anthropophilic dermatophytes are more common in the community. In some cases there is evidence to support the existence of localized epidemics

Dermatophyte species		
Anthropophilic species	**Zoophilic species**	**Geophilic species**
E. floccosum		
T. rubrum	*T. mentagrophytes*	
T. mentagrophytes var. *interdigitale*	var. *mentagrophytes*	
	T. erinacei	
T. tonsurans	*T. verrucosum*	
T. soudanense	*T. equinum*	
T. violacum	*T. quinckeanum*	
T. schoenleinii	*T. simii*	
T. concentricum		
T. megninii		
T. gourvilii		
T. yaoundei		
M. audouinii	*M. canis*	*M. gypseum*
M. rivalieri	*M. persicolor*	*M. fulvum*
M. ferrugineum	*M. equinum*	
	M. nanum	
	M. gallinae	

↑ **Fig. 12**
Dermatophyte species.

of infection where there are appropriate conditions for transmission. These are seen in swimming pools, school changing areas and industrial shower rooms where infected skin scales can be shed on wet floors. Spread of dermatophytosis of the feet has led to a heavy rate of infection among coal miners in Europe where, in some mines, the infection rate is 35% or more. Bacterial foot infection is also common in this group and may follow dermatophytosis. Nail infections caused by dermatophytes are common, and studies from the UK suggest that about 2.7% of the population have onychomycosis with an incidence of infection approaching 5 per 1000 each year. At least 50% of these do not present for treatment.

Tinea capitis caused by anthropophilic organisms is sporadic in incidence. In Asia and Africa, certain urban areas in the USA and in the UK, epidemics of this infection have been described affecting numbers of children. Transmission can occur following brief contact with an infected child.

In most surveys of dermatophyte infections the dominant species is *Trichophyton rubrum*. However, the relative incidence of the different species varies according to the geographic location, particularly where scalp infections are common, and has been known to change over time.

Mycology

The dermatophytes are identified almost entirely by studying their morphology. The classification of the three genera is traditionally based on features of the macroconidia. In *Trichophyton* they are cylindrical and smooth-walled (see Fig. 26); in *Epidermophyton* they are club-shaped with walls becoming slightly rough (see Fig. 30); and in *Microsporum* species they are generally fusiform and rough-walled (see Fig. 34). A number of species, however, do not produce macroconidia. These are assigned to the genera by considering other characteristics which demonstrate their taxonomic affinities. There are a few physiologic tests which can be employed to aid in dermatophyte identification.

Clinical features and agents of infection

Dermatophyte infections are normally called 'tinea' followed by the Latin name of the appropriate part of the body involved. A body lesion is therefore tinea corporis; other forms include tinea pedis, tinea cruris, tinea capitis and tinea facei. The classical appearance of ringworm is the round scaly lesion where the rim is more inflamed and scaly than the center; this occurs in body infections and is known as tinea circinata (**Fig. 13**). Nail infections, tinea unguium, may also be described as onychomycosis due to dermatophytes. Tinea incognito indicates an atypical presentation of a dermatophyte infection, usually associated with the inappropriate therapeutic use of topical corticosteroids.

Tinea pedis, tinea manuum, tinea unguium and tinea curis

Tinea pedis is the most frequently occuring dermatophyte infection and is caused by anthropophilic fungi such as *Trichophyton rubrum, T. mentagrophytes* var. *interdigitale (T. interdigitale)* and less frequently by *Epidermophyton floccosum.* The earliest lesion develops with scaling and itching between the toes, particularly the lateral third and fourth interdigital spaces (**Fig. 14**); this may spread to the undersurface of the toes.

Other presentations of tinea pedis include the chronic 'dry type' or 'moccasin' infections where the soles are covered with a dry scaly rash usually caused by *T. rubrum* (**Fig. 15**), and also the inflammatory conditions with blisters on the soles or under the toes which are generally only seen with *T. interdigitale* (**Fig. 16**). In chronic cases, erosion of the skin of the toe webs may enlarge with the appearance of a greenish discoloration due to the presence of Gram-negative bacteria such as *Pseudomonas* (dermatophytosis complex) (**Fig. 17**), which may replace the dermatophyte.

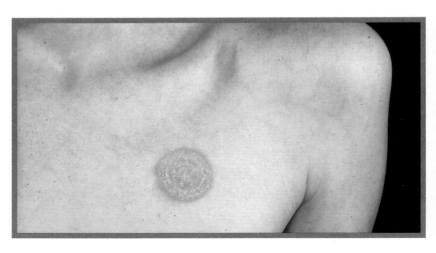

↑ **Fig. 13**
Tinea circinata (ringworm).

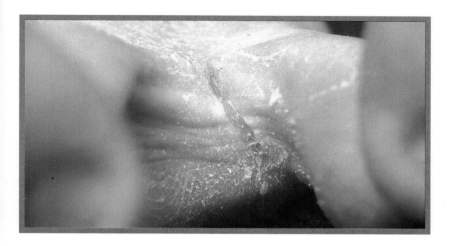

↑ **Fig. 14**
Tinea pedis. Interdigital scaling.

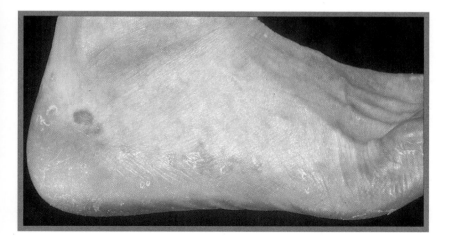

↑ **Fig. 15**
Tinea pedis. Dry-type infection.

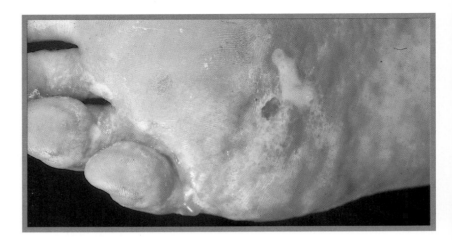

↑ Fig. 16
Tinea pedis. Inflammatory lesion showing blisters.

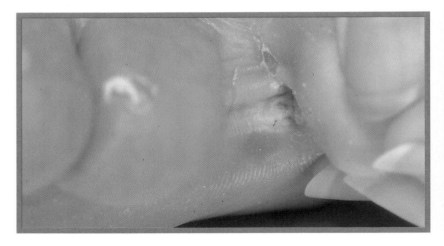

↑ Fig. 17
Tinea pedis. Complication with Gram-negative infection.

Tinea manuum. Dry-type dermatophytosis affecting the palms caused by *T. rubrum* may accompany foot infections. The palm is covered with fine scales (**Fig. 18**) and there may be involvement of the finger nails. Itching is generally minimal. The involvement of one hand and both feet is typical and suggestive of this condition, although bilateral palmar infections may also occur. Other dermatophytes may affect the palm or dorsum of the hand, particularly if there is a disease of keratinization such as palmar–plantar keratoderma. This form of infection has to be distinguished from eczema and psoriasis.

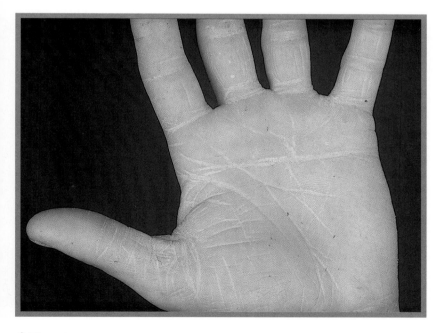

↑ **Fig. 18**
Tinea manuum.

Tinea unguium (onychomycosis). This is an infection of the nail plate. In the case of dermatophytes the usual causes are anthropophilic organisms. Dermatophytes usually invade the nail from the distal and lateral margins when the first change is separation of the nail plate from its bed – onycholysis. Subsequently they produce a thickened, discolored and broken nail. Onychomycosis is more frequent in the toenails than the fingers and usually the whole nail plate is involved and dystrophic (**Fig. 19**). Generally the adjacent skin is also infected. Dermatophyte onychomycosis is rare in children.

The causative organisms of tinea unguium are:
- *T. rubrum*
- *T. interdigitale*
- Rarely, other dermatophytes, particularly those which cause scalp infections.

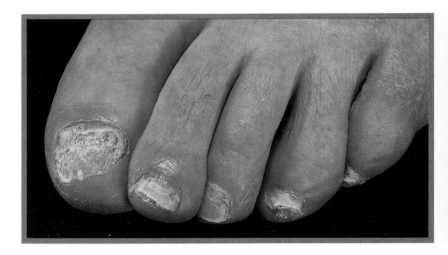

↑ **Fig. 19**
Tinea unguium due to *Trichophyton rubrum*.

Infection with *T. rubrum*, the most frequent pathogen, can involve several nails of toes and fingers showing distal and lateral subungual onychomycosis to total nail infection. This often coexists with dry-type infections of the hands and feet.

T. interdigitale infection occurs less frequently, mainly involving a great toe nail, and can be secondary to other forms of nail dystrophy such as onychogryphosis. It is a cause of superficial white onychomycosis.

Other dermatophytes may invade nails, causing pitting, transverse ridges and splitting of the nail plate surface.

The characteristic clinical syndrome of rapid onset proximal subungual onychomycosis is particularly associated with AIDS patients.

The features of onychomycosis due to different groups of fungi are shown in **Figure 20**.

Differential diagnosis of onychomycosis			
Dermatophyte	*Candida*	*Scytalidium*	**Other molds**
Site			
Toenails	Fingernails	Toenails	Usually a single toenail
Fingernails		Finger nails	
Signs			
Thickening	Onycholysis	Dystrophy	Thickening
Discoloration	Paronychia	Paronychia	Dystrophy
Skin lesions			
Feet, palms	None	Feet, palms	None

↑ **Fig. 20**
Differential diagnosis of onychomycosis.

Tinea cruris presents with scaling in the groin extending to the upper surface of the thigh and around the perineum, often with a raised margin. It is mainly seen in adult men (**Fig. 21**). The infection is generally bilateral and itchy. The fungi involved are *T. rubrum, T. interdigitale* and *Epidermophyton floccosum*. Other causes of groin rash include candidosis and erythrasma. Flexural psoriasis may also produce scaling in this area with erythematous and soggy skin, but usually there are psoriatic lesions at other sites such as the umbilicus.

Description of species
Of the species causing tinea pedis, onychomycosis and tinea cruris, *Trichophyton rubrum* is by far the most prevalent. *T. mentagrophytes* var. *interdigitale* and *Epidermophyton floccosum* are also involved.

T. rubrum has a variable morphology. The most frequently occurring form has white floccose colonies with a dark red to brown pigment on the reverse (**Fig. 22**). Some isolates produce a melanoid pigment which diffuses throughout the medium and colors the entire plate (**Fig. 23**). Under the microscope the microconidia can be numerous or scanty. They are oval in shape and are borne along the sides of the hyphae (**Fig. 24**).

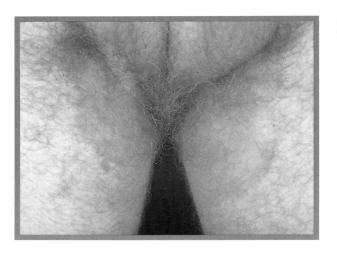

← **Fig. 21
Tinea cruris.**

→ Fig. 22
Trichophyton rubrum colonies showing the typical form.

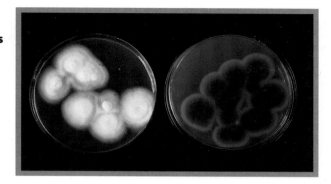

→ Fig. 23
Trichophyton rubrum. Melanoid colonies.

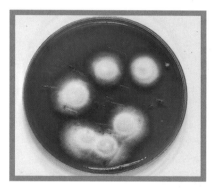

→ Fig. 24
Trichophyton rubrum microconidia.

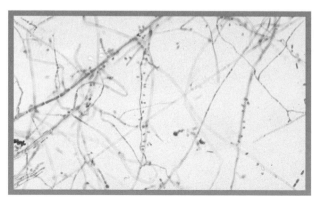

A granular form of *T. rubrum* is occasionally isolated which has a coarse, folded surface (**Fig. 25**). The picture on microscopy is quite unlike that of the typical form of the species and shows numerous macroconidia (**Fig. 26**).

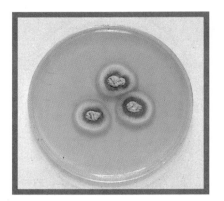

← **Fig. 25**
Colonies of the granular form of *Trichophyton rubrum*.

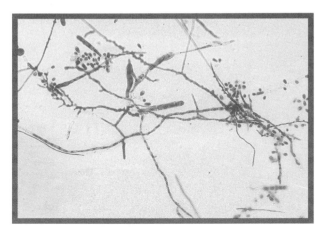

← **Fig. 26**
Macroconidia of granular *Trichophyton rubrum*.

T. mentagrophytes var. *interdigitale* produces white floccose colonies which become cream colored and powdery in the center as the conidia develop (**Fig. 27**). There are abundant microconidia which are spherical in shape and are borne in clusters as well as along the hyphae. Macroconidia, which are cylindrical and smooth walled, may be present. Spiral hyphae are frequently seen (**Fig. 28**).

→ Fig. 27
Trichophyton mentagrophytes
var. *interdigitale* colonies.

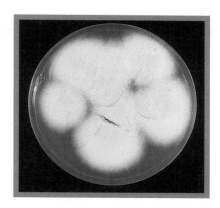

→ Fig. 28
Microscopy of
Trichophyton
mentagro-
phytes var.
interdigitale.

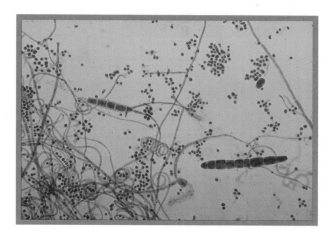

Epidermophyton floccosum has colonies that develop quickly and have a dull green or khaki-colored, powdery surface. As the culture ages the surface may become folded and white floccose patches appear (**Fig. 29**). Pyriform, slightly rough-walled macroconidia are formed early and these are diagnostic of the species (**Fig. 30**). No microconidia are produced, but numerous chlamydospores may be present, particularly in old cultures.

Tinea corporis
Tinea corporis may be caused by either zoophilic fungi or anthropophilic organisms, less frequently by geophilic fungi. Lesions are annular, often irregular and may be multiple. The edge is usually clearly seen and the hair follicles are prominent (**Fig. 31**). Generally, in infections caused by zoophilic dermatophytes the lesions are inflamed and itch severely. With anthropophilic fungi such as *Trichophyton rubrum* the lesions are often large and have a

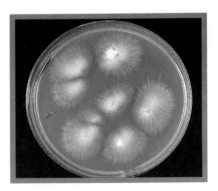

← **Fig. 29**
Colonies of *Epidermophyton floccosum*.

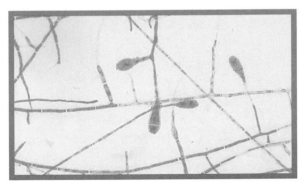

← **Fig. 30**
Microscopy of *Epidermophyton floccosum*.

poorly defined border with less erythema or scaling (**Fig. 32**).

The most frequent causes of tinea corporis of animal origin are *Microsporum canis, T. verrucosum, T. mentagrophytes* var. *mentagrophytes* and *T. erinacei*. Other species met are *M. persicolor, M. equinum* and *T. equinum*. The geophilic species seen occasionally is *M. gypseum*.

→ Fig. 31
Tinea corporis
due to
Microsporum
gypseum.

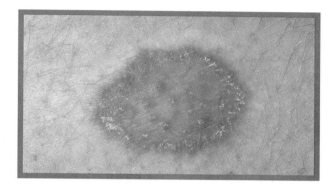

→ Fig. 32
Tinea corporis due to
Trichophyton rubrum.

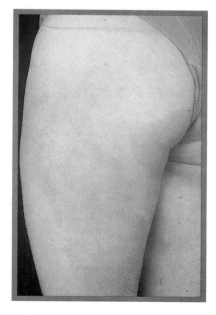

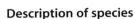

Description of species

Microsporum canis causes infections in cats and dogs. It produces rapidly growing colonies which have a flat surface with abundant aerial hyphae. The center becomes buff colored with age. There is a yellow to orange pigment on reverse (**Fig. 33**). The fusiform, rough-walled macroconidia are diagnostic of the species (**Fig. 34**).

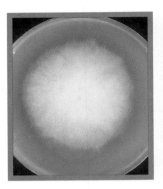
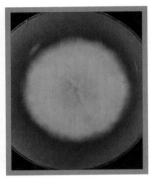

← **Fig. 33**
Colonies of
Microsporum
canis.

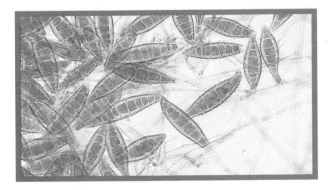

← **Fig. 34**
Macroconidia of
Microsporum
canis.

A glabrous form of *M. canis* is occasionally encountered with colonies that are waxy in texture and feathery in appearance and with much submerged growth at the edge (**Fig. 35**). These isolates are unstable and revert to the typical form with age.

Trichophyton verrucosum is the agent of cattle ringworm. The white colonies are very slow growing and have a hard texture (**Fig. 36**). Growth in culture is faster at 37°C than at 26°C. Micro- and macroconidia are absent but chlamydospores are produced (**Fig. 37**) and these are particularly numerous at 37°C.

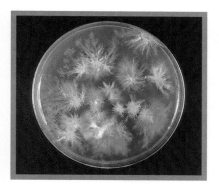

← Fig. 35
Glabrous colonies of
Microsporum canis.

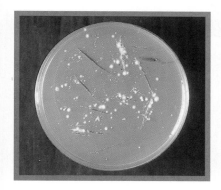

↑ Fig. 36
Slow-growing hard colonies of
Trichophyton verrucosum.

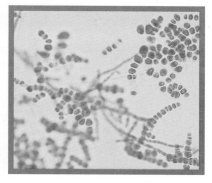

↑ Fig. 37
Microscopy of *Trichophyton*
verrucosum.

Trichophyton mentagrophytes var. *mentagrophytes* infects a range of domestic, farm and wild animals, usually rodents. The colonies have a white or cream powdery, granular surface with a radiate margin. A red or brown pigment often develops on the reverse (**Fig. 38**). There are numerous spherical microconidia which are borne in clusters as well as along the sides of the hyphae. Smooth-walled, cylindrical macroconidia may be present as well as spiral hyphae (**Fig. 39**).

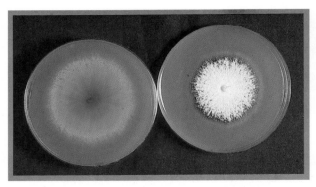

← **Fig. 38**
Colony of
Trichophyton
mentagrophytes
var.
mentagrophytes.

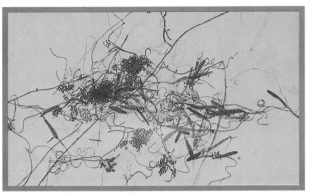

← **Fig. 39**
Microscopy of
Trichophyton
mentagrophytes
var.
mentagrophytes.

Trichophyton erinacei is the cause of hedgehog ringworm in the UK and New Zealand. It produces rapidly growing colonies with a white powdery surface and a bright yellow pigment on the reverse (**Fig. 40**). There are numerous elongated microconidia borne along the hyphae (**Fig. 41**). This species can be distinguished physiologically from *T. mentagrophytes* by demonstrating its inability to attack urea.

→ Fig. 40 Colony of *Trichophyton erinacei*.

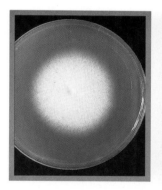
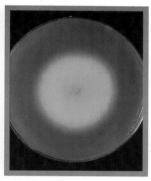

→ Fig. 41 Microscopy of *Trichophyton erinacei*.

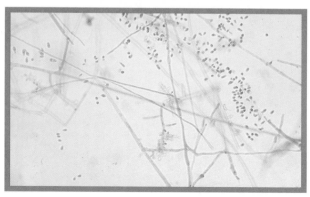

Microsporum persicolor is associated with small rodents, especially voles, and is occasionally a cause of infection in man. The colonies develop rapidly to produce a thick surface texture with a powdery appearance in the center. The color on both aspects may be white, cream or pink (**Fig. 42**). It can be distinguished from *Trichophyton mentagrophytes* by its production of a deep pink surface color on 1% peptone agar. Numerous microconidia are formed, but the slender fusiform macroconidia with slightly roughened walls at the tip are typical of the species (**Fig. 43**).

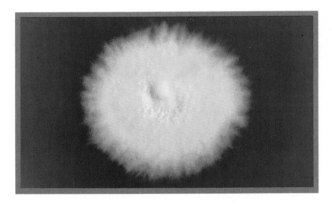

← **Fig. 42
Colony of
*Microsporum
persicolor.***

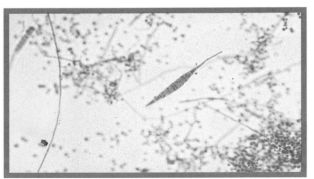

← **Fig. 43
Microscopy of
*Microsporum
persicolor.***

M. gypseum is a geophilic species which develops rapidly growing colonies with a buff-colored, powdery surface texture (**Fig. 44**). Both micro- and macroconidia are formed, but the morphology of the numerous macroconidia is characteristic of the species. They are fusiform but with blunt ends and the walls are roughened and thin (**Fig. 45**).

→ Fig. 44
Colonies of *Microsporum gypseum*.

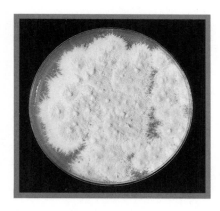

→ Fig. 45
Microscopy of *Microsporum gypseum*.

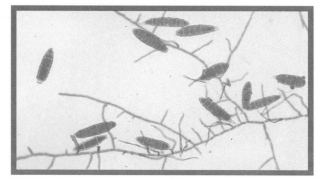

Tinea capitis

Tinea capitis (scalp ringworm) usually presents in childhood with patches of scalp hair loss and scaling. There is a background of erythema, although in some children this is minimal (**Fig. 46**). The intensity of inflammation varies: the zoophilic fungi usually produce more crusting and suppuration. At its most extreme this type of inflammatory lesion affecting a hair-bearing area is boggy and pustular, known as kerion, which is an inflammatory response to the dermatophyte itself rather than a secondary bacterial infection (**Fig. 47**). Hair loss is seldom permanent unless an extensive kerion forms, and even then there is a surprising degree of recovery. The severity of itching is variable.

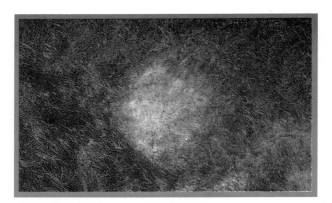

← **Fig. 46
Tinea capitis.**

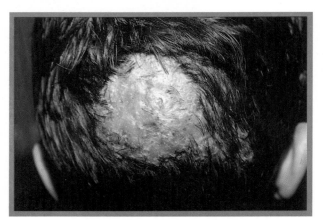

← **Fig. 47
Kerion.**

There are three main patterns of hair infection which are classified according to the location of the majority of the fungal spores once the dermatophyte has invaded the hair shaft. They are ectothrix, endothrix and favic and are detected by careful microscopic examination of infected hairs. The patterns, in part, determine the site of breakage of hairs and the clinical appearances. Some preliminary help with the diagnosis can also be obtained by shining a filtered ultraviolet light (Wood's light) on the lesions. *Microsporum*, but not *Trichophyton*, species fluoresce green when viewed with this light in a darkened room (**Fig. 48**). An exception is favus, caused by *Trichophyton schoenleinii*, when the hairs have a dull green fluorescence. The Wood's light can also be used to identify infected hairs for culture.

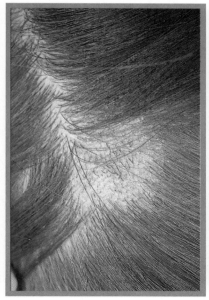
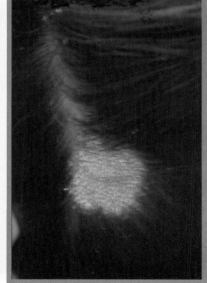

↑ **Fig. 48**
Fluorescent tinea capitis.

With *Microsporum*-infected hairs there is a small-spored ectothrix arrangement. Although invasion starts inside the hair shaft, most of the fungus is outside the hair, forming a sheath of spores (**Fig. 49**). In endothrix hairs caused by *Trichophyton* species, the spores are contained entirely inside the hair (**Fig. 50**).

Although the clinical and microscopic features of scalp infections will indicate a probable source of infection, the final decision rests with the results of culture. An endothrix infection will always indicate a pathogen of anthropophilic origin and in the USA it is this type of infection, due to *T. tonsurans*, which predominates. Endothrix infections are currently frequent in the UK and, although *T. tonsurans* is again responsible for the majority, a number of species have been isolated in recent years.

The zoophilic *Microsporum canis,* which produces fluorescing hairs with an ectothrix arrangement of spores, has been a major source of scalp infection in the UK in the past and is prominent in Mediterranean countries and North Africa. Ectothrix-infected hairs which do not fluoresce are characteristic of zoophilic *Trichophyton* species such as *T. verrucosum* (**Fig. 51**). The spores are larger than those seen in hairs infected by *Microsporum* species.

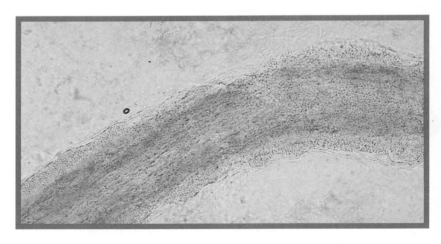

↑ **Fig. 49**
Hair showing a small-spored ectothrix infection caused by
Microsporum canis.

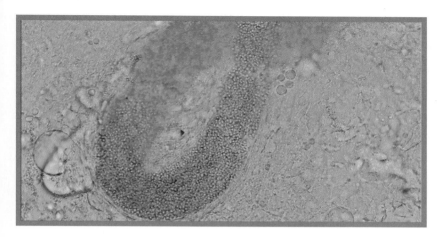

↑ Fig. 50
Hair showing an endothrix infection caused by *Trichophyton tonsurans*.

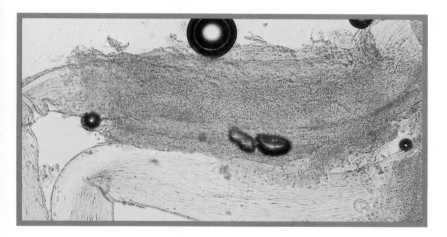

↑ Fig. 51
Large-spored ectothrix infection of hair infected by *Trichophyton verrucosum*.

Favus is now a rare infection seen in small foci in the USA, North Africa and the Middle East. It is clinically important as it may present with multiple crusts or scutula in the scalp (**Fig. 52**), causing scarring alopecia and it will affect adults (mainly women) in addition to children. The hairs are not as heavily infected as those with the endothrix pattern shown by *T. tonsurans* and they continue to grow to form long lengths of infected hair. Air spaces can be seen between the hyphae when the hairs are first placed in KOH (**Fig. 53**).

A summary of the features of tinea capitis is given in **Figure 54**.

Scalp scaling without hair loss occurs in a number of other conditions. In children seborrheic dermatitis, psoriasis or pityriasis amiantacea may have a similar appearance. In the last of these conditions copious thick scales are present around hairs. In alopecia areata, where there are patches of hair loss, there is usually no scaling and small numbers of broken tapering hairs (exclamation mark hairs) can be seen.

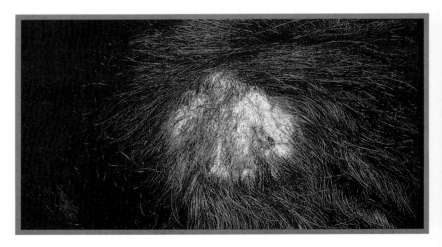

↑ Fig. 52
Favus.

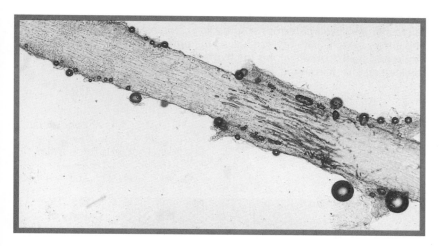

↑ Fig. 53
Hair from a case of favus showing the presence of hyphae and air spaces.

Features of tinea capitis

Organism	Hair invasion	Wood's light	Source
Microsporum canis	Ectothrix	Positive	Cat, dog
M. audouinii	Ectothrix	Positive	Man
M. rivalieri	Ectothrix	Positive	Man
Trichophyton tonsurans	Endothrix	Negative	Man
T. violaceum	Endothrix	Negative	Man
T. soudanense	Endothrix	Negative	Man
T. schoenleinii	Favic	Positive	Man
T. verrucosum	Ectothrix	Negative	Cattle

↑ Fig. 54
The features of tinea capitis.

Description of species

Microsporum audouinii forms flat spreading colonies with thin surface growth and a silky texture. The reverse has a pink pigment (**Fig. 55**). There may be elongated microconidia along the hyphae and if macroconidia are present they are distorted in shape (**Fig. 56**).

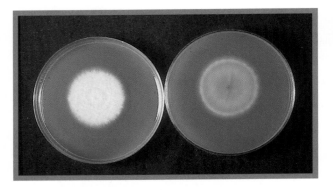

← **Fig. 55
Colony of
*Microsporum
audouinii*.**

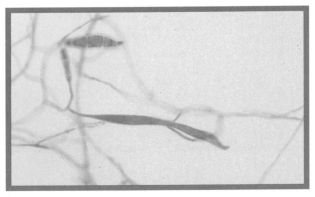

← **Fig. 56
Microscopy of
*Microsporum
audouinii*.**

M. rivalieri is a variant of *M. audouinii* and produces white folded colonies with a matt texture resembling ground glass (**Fig. 57**). The characteristic feature on microscopy is the presence of comb-like projections on the hyphae known as pectinate hyphae (**Fig. 58**).

→ Fig. 57
Colonies of *Microsporum rivalieri*.

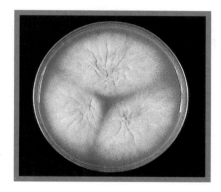

→ Fig. 58
Microscopy of *Microsporum rivalieri*.

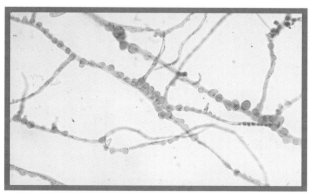

Trichophyton tonsurans develops powdery colonies which become folded as the culture ages. The surface color can be white, gray, buff or yellow (**Fig. 59**). There is usually a dark brown pigment on the reverse. The microconidia are numerous and variable in size, borne along the hyphae and on short side branches forming loose clusters. Chlamydospores are common but smooth-walled macroconidia and spiral hyphae are infrequently observed (**Fig. 60**).

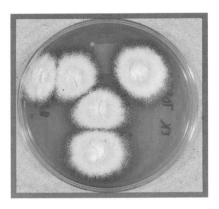

**← Fig. 59
Colonies of *Trichophyton tonsurans*.**

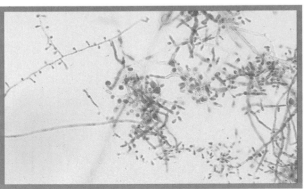

**← Fig. 60
Microscopy of *Trichophyton tonsurans*.**

T. soudanense produces slow-growing glabrous colonies with a soft or brittle texture and a prominent stellate fringe. The color is orange but many isolates develop a deep red color with age (**Fig. 61**). Microconidia may be present along the hyphae, but the typical feature on microscopy is the reflexive branching on hyphae composed of short segments (**Fig. 62**).

→ Fig. 61
Colonies of *Trichophyton soudanense*.

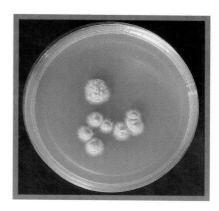

→ Fig. 62
Microscopy of *Trichophyton soudanense*.

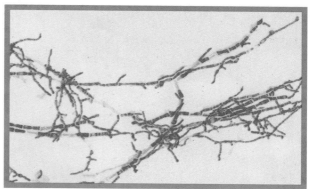

T. violaceum has glabrous colonies which are slow-growing and hard in texture. They are deep red in color (**Fig. 63**). Micro- and macroconidia are rare or absent (**Fig. 64**).

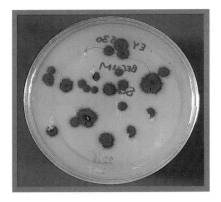

← **Fig. 63**
Colonies of *Trichophyton violaceum*.

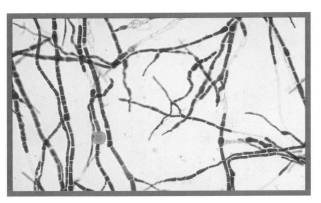

← **Fig. 64**
Microscopy of *Trichophyton violaceum*.

T. schoenleinii colonies are slow-growing with a glabrous texture. The color is white or gray, the surface rough and convoluted, and there is considerable submerged growth around the edge of the colony (**Fig. 65**). The important feature on microscopy is the presence of 'antler-like' hyphae where the tips of the hyphal branches are rounded and swollen (**Fig. 66**). There are no micro- or macroconidia.

→ Fig. 65
Colonies of *Trichophyton schoenleinii*.

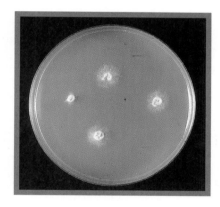

→ Fig. 66
Microscopy of *Trichophyton schoenleinii*.

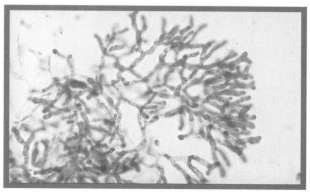

Other sites for dermatophyte infection

Tinea facei or ringworm of the face is uncommon but may be difficult to recognize as it presents with erythema, scaling and soreness. The typical annular rim is difficult to see but may be found in the preauricular and submental regions. Facial tinea may also flare in sunlight.

Tinea barbae or facial tinea affecting the neck and beard area is usually highly inflammatory and caused by a zoophilic fungus such as *T. verrucosum*. Again the annular shape may be difficult to recognize and the rash may be pustular without much scaling (**Fig. 67**). It is difficult to distinguish from staphylococcal infection in this site but there is usually less scaling with the latter. Culture will establish the correct diagnosis.

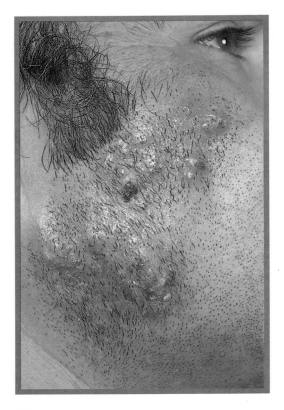

← **Fig. 67**
Tinea barbae.

Tinea incognito (steroid-modified tinea), following the application of potent corticosteroids to a dermatophyte infection, usually results in loss of scaling and annular rim, reduction of itch and the formation of prominent pustules or papules (**Fig. 68**). After long-term application, however, other corticosteroid-induced side effects such as striae and bruising may be apparent. There is no evidence, however, that a cream containing a hydrocortisone/steroid combination can cause similar changes.

→ Fig. 68
Tinea incognito.

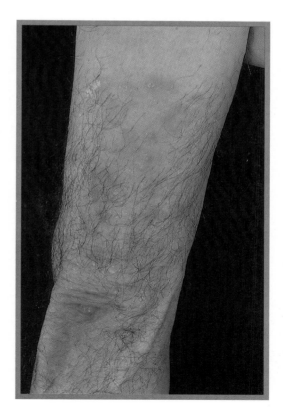

Tinea imbricata is the name given to an exotic infection caused by *T. concentricum* which is found in the west Pacific, Southeast Asia and Amazonia. It may be very common in endemic areas within the tropical rain forest but is seldom seen elsewhere. It is characterized by extensive and persistent rings of concentric scales (**Fig. 69**). The colonies of *T. concentricum* are slow growing and glabrous with a soft texture. The color is gray or buff (**Fig. 70**). There are hyphal swellings and chlamydospores on microscopy but micro- and macroconidia are absent or rare.

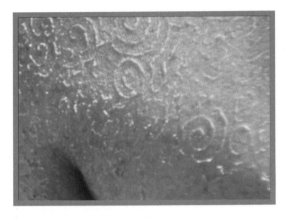

← **Fig. 69**
Tinea imbricata.

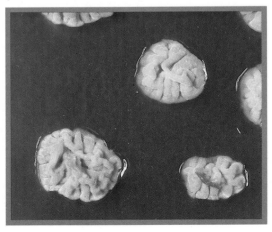

← **Fig. 70**
Colonies of
Trichophyton
concentricum.

Majocchi's granuloma describes the late stage of a hair shaft invasion, where occasionally a persistent granuloma, often without visible or viable fungi, remains within the skin. It is often caused by *T. rubrum.* (**Fig. 71**).

**→ Fig. 71
Majocchi's granuloma.**

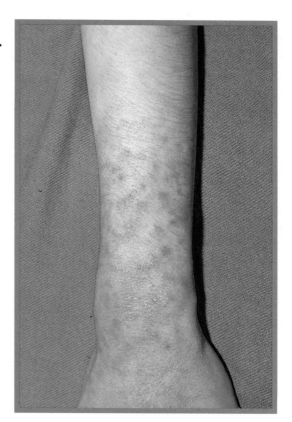

Dermatophyte id or dermatophytide reactions

Id reactions are inflammatory conditions of the skin which do not contain fungi but are an allergic reaction to a dermatophyte infection. They often appear to be precipitated by treatment of dermatophytosis. The commonest forms are acute vesicular eczema of the hands or feet (pompholyx) associated with inflammatory tinea pedis caused by *Trichophyton interdigitale* and a disseminated papular rash associated with inflammatory tinea corporis or capitis. Other id reactions include erythema nodosum and multiforme. Generally such patients have very strong delayed type skin test reactions to dermatophyte antigens but the immunologic basis of the dermatophyte id reaction is unknown.

Additional tests used in the identification of dermatophytes show:
- presence of urease,
- penetration of hair *in vitro*,
- growth on rice grains,
- pigment production on 1% peptone agar
- nutritional requirements.

The urea agar base (Difco) used to test for the presence of urease is prepared in solid form and dispensed in tubes or bottles. A change in the color of the medium from yellow to red within 7 days indicates the ability to attack urea. This distinguishes *Trichophyton rubrum* and *T. erinacei* (both negative) from *T. mentagrophytes* (positive) (**Fig. 72**).

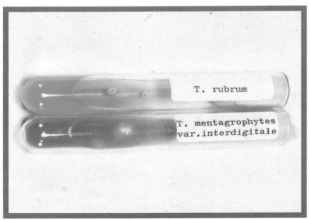

← **Fig. 72**
Urease test showing *Trichophyton rubrum* as negative; *T. mentagrophytes* as positive.

The ability to form transverse perforations in sterile hair *in vitro* will distinguish T. *rubrum* from T. *mentagrophytes*. Short lengths of human hair are sterilized and added to dilute yeast extract in a Petri dish. After inoculation the hairs are incubated for up to 2 weeks and examined for the formation of wedge-shaped perforations which are produced by T. *mentagrophytes* (**Fig. 73**). No perforations are formed by T. *rubrum*.

Testing for growth on rice is performed by placing a few grains in a small flask or bottle, covering them with distilled water and autoclaving. The fungus is inoculated onto the surface of the grains and incubated for 7–14 days. This test distinguishes *Microsporum audouinii*, which will not grow on the rice grains, from *M. canis* and *M. gypseum*, both of which produce thick growth (**Fig. 74**).

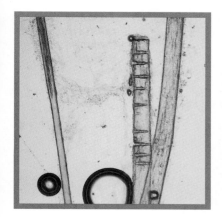

↑ **Fig. 73**
Hair penetration by
Trichophyton mentagrophytes.

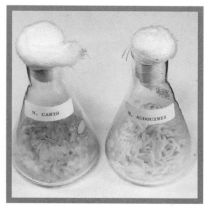

↑ **Fig. 74**
Growth on rice grains by
***Microsporum canis;* no growth**
by *M. audouinii.*

M. persicolor develops a pink color on the surface of the colony after 7–14 days when grown on agar containing 1% peptone. No pigment is formed by *Trichophyton mentagrophytes* (**Fig. 75**).

The series of *Trichophyton* agars Nos 1–7 (Difco) can be used to differentiate some *Trichophyton* species by demonstrating the requirement for growth factors. Examples are *T. equinum*, which requires nicotinic acid, and *T. tonsurans*, which requires thiamine.

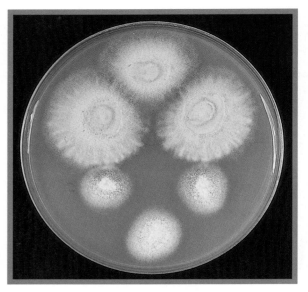

← **Fig. 75**
***Microsporum persicolor* (top) and *Trichophyton mentagrophytes* (bottom) on 1% peptone agar.**

The management of dermatophytosis

Topical therapy. The simple principle for therapy is that topical treatment is generally used if the infection is not widespread and does not involve either hair or nails. For most superficial infections caused by dermatophytes, a topical imidazole, tolnaftate, terbinafine, amorolfine or cyclopiroxolamine is adequate. The minimum treatment period has never been clearly established but, as a general rule, the specific antifungal agents clear tinea cruris/corporis within 2 weeks. Benzoic acid (Whitfield's ointment) takes longer, about 4 weeks. However, terbinafine may take much less time, 7 days.

In tinea pedis of the dry type, most topical agents take 4 weeks to produce a remission and the relapse rate is high.

In nail disease there is evidence that some agents, eg tioconazole, amorolfine, cyclopiroxolamine, may occasionally produce a cure, although success rates are still comparatively low.

Topical therapy is not indicated for treatment of scalp infections.

Oral therapy. Itraconazole is given at doses of 400mg daily for tinea cruris/corporis (1 week) and tinea pedis (1–2 weeks). For nail infections it is given at doses of 400mg daily for 1 week every month for 2–4 months.

Ketoconazole (200mg daily) is effective in treating dermatophytosis. However, in view of the rare complication of hepatitis in 1:10,000 cases it has largely been superseded by itraconazole, even though the main risk of this complication followed long-term therapy for nail disease.

Fluconazole is available in a few countries for the treatment of dermatophytosis in doses of 50–100mg daily or 150mg weekly.

Terbinafine is used in doses of 250mg daily for a wide range of dermatophyte infections. For tinea cruris/corporis and dry-type foot infections it is given for 2 weeks. Terbinafine produces better results than griseofulvin in the therapy of nail disease. The optimum duration of therapy for onychomycosis is about 6 weeks for finger nails and 3 months for toe nails.

Griseofulvin is used for dermatophytosis of the skin, dry-type tinea pedis and scalp and nail disease. Remission rates are lower than with either the oral azoles, ketoconazole and itraconazole, or with terbinafine for dry-type *Trichophyton rubrum* infections and for nail disease. However, for certain scalp infections such as those caused by *Microsporum canis* it is the most appropriate therapy. The dose of griseofulvin is 10mg/kg daily. It should be given for at least 6 weeks in tinea capitis. Long-term success rates in onychomycosis affecting the toenails are less than 40%, although the results in fingernail infections are considerably better.

4.2 Superficial candidosis

Infections caused by yeasts of the genus *Candida* frequently affect the mucous membranes or the skin. The principal pathogen is *Candida albicans*, although other species such as *C. tropicalis, C. parapsilosis, C. krusei* and *C. glabrata* may also cause human infections.

Candida species are normal commensals in the mouth, gastrointestinal tract and vaginal mucosa; they are less frequently isolated from healthy skin. Superficial *Candida* infections are worldwide in occurrence although there are some regional differences in the prevalence of patterns of infection. Interdigital candidosis of the feet is more common in the tropics whereas onychomycosis without paronychia due to *Candida* is mainly seen in colder climates. Numerous factors are known to predispose to candidosis (see Fig. 4) and it is generally possible to find an underlying reason for infection. A common exception to this is vaginal candidosis, where most women with this condition have no detectable predisposition. Although it may affect all ages, infants and the elderly are particularly susceptible to superficial candidosis, which probably reflects the immaturity or senescence of their immune responses.

Most *Candida* infections are endogenous, the key event being a change in the relationship between the yeast and host. The process of infection starts with adherence of commensal organisms to mucosal cells or keratinocytes, which probably involves the interaction of a fungal cell wall polysaccharide with a human receptor site on an epithelial cell.

Pathology
In the early stages of *Candida* invasion the main changes are the infiltration of the epithelium by neutrophils with some hyper- and parakeratosis. There is an upper dermal infiltrate of lymphocytes and plasma cells. Dysplastic changes of the epithelium may develop in some chronic infections of the oral mucosa, which raises the possibility that persistent oral candidosis, either on its own or in combination with some other factor, such as smoking, may lead to the development of oral squamous carcinomas.

Clinical features
Superficial candidosis principally affects the body sites which support carriage of the organism, such as the mouth or vagina, but it may also affect the skin or nails. Infections of the skin generally involve body fold areas. Cutaneous manifestations of systemic candidosis will be discussed later.

Oral candidosis.

Oral candidosis, or thrush, is a common infection of the elderly, denture wearers, infants and immunocompromised patients. It is the most frequently occurring infectious complication of AIDS. There are a number of different clinical types of oropharyngeal candidosis which can be largely distinguished by their chronicity and clinical appearance:

- acute pseudomembranous candidosis (**Fig. 76**), which presents with white, easily detached plaques on the inflamed epithelium;

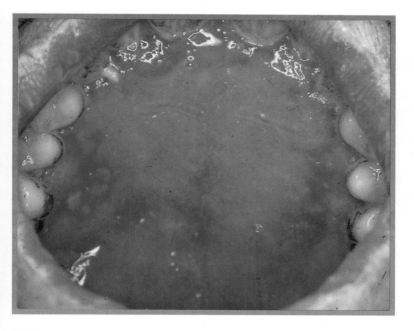

↑ **Fig. 76**
Acute pseudomembranous candidosis.

- chronic pseudomembranous candidosis (**Fig. 77**), a persistent condition often seen in AIDS which is refractory to therapy;
- acute erythematous candidosis (acute atrophic oral candidosis), where plaques are not formed but the mucosal surface appears red and glazed;
- chronic erythematous candidosis, characterized by persistent erythema and occurring in patients presenting with inflammatory changes and oral discomfort associated with dentures (denture sore mouth);
- chronic plaque-like candidosis (**Fig. 78**), having the appearance of a white plaque on the tongue and other areas of the mouth, which cannot be detached;

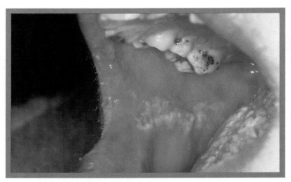

← **Fig. 77**
Chronic pseudomembranous candidosis.

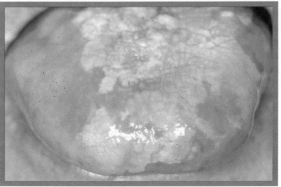

← **Fig. 78**
Chronic plaque-like candidosis.

- chronic nodular candidosis, where the mucosa has a pebbly appearance;
- angular cheilitis (**Fig. 79**), which can accompany any of the above changes;
- median rhomboid glossitis, taking the form of a chronic lozenge-shaped area of *Candida* infection on the dorsal surface of the tongue.

Although the features of chronic erythematous candidosis are related to the presence of *Candida*, treatment of the yeast alone will not control the condition and the addition of oral antiseptics is usually necessary, suggesting that oral bacteria may also play a role. Chronic plaque-like candidosis may be an additional feature found in smokers with chronic candidosis. Histologically it contains epithelial atypia and, in some patients, oral carcinomas have subsequently developed. The characteristic splitting at the corners of the mouth in angular cheilitis is an important and common sign of candidosis and can be spotted easily.

In most patients with oral candidosis the main focus of infection is on the buccal mucosa, but in severely infected individuals there is involvement of the tongue or pharynx, as well as the esophagus. Esophageal candidosis is mainly seen in patients with AIDS, leukemia or chronic mucocutaneous candidosis. While it may present with retrosternal pain on swallowing it is often silent.

Secondary oral infection due to *Candida* may occur in subjects with epithelial abnormalities such as hyperkeratosis or ulceration and in conditions such as lichen planus, pemphigus and white sponge nevus.

→ Fig. 79 Angular cheilitis.

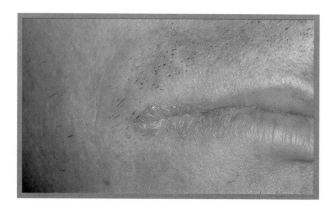

Vaginal candidosis

Vaginal *Candida* infection is normally caused by *C. albicans* although other *Candida* species such as *C. glabrata* or *C. tropicalis* have also been implicated. Although it occurs in pregnant women or diabetics, one of the features of this condition is that there is usually no underlying abnormality to be found. Theories about the causes of vaginal candidosis include the use of tampons, tightly fitting underwear and immunologic deficiencies. However, severely immunocompromised women do not usually show a higher incidence of persistent vaginal infections than appropriate control groups. The main clinical forms of vaginal candidosis are given in **Figure 80**.

The symptoms of all forms are similar, with the appearance of itching and discharge. Vaginal pain and dyspareunia may also occur. The clinical appearance varies with the presence or absence of soft white plaques (thrush). The course of infection is unpredictable and although most women have a single episode of infection others may have either recurrent attacks or persistent thrush. No clear reasons for these are apparent, although patients with recurrent symptoms have been found to have a higher incidence of familial atopic diseases such as hay fever or asthma, suggesting that sensitization may play a role in the development of symptoms. Women on high-dose estrogen replacement therapy may also have more frequent episodes of vaginal candidosis.

Secondary candidosis may occur in those with underlying mucosal disease such as pemphigoid, lichen planus or Behçet's syndrome.

Clinical forms of vaginal candidosis

Acute (pseudomembranous or erythematous) vaginal candidosis

Chronic relapsing vaginal candidosis

Persistent vaginal candidosis

Secondary vaginal candidosis

↑ **Fig. 80**
Clinical forms of vaginal candidosis.

Candida intertrigo

The skin is only indirectly involved in vaginal candidosis when there is spread of infection to the vulva and the perineum. In this case a prominent red rash in the groin and on the upper surface of the thighs may appear with satellite pustules and papules (**Fig. 81**). The same can occur in other sites such as under the breasts and in the umbilicus. In some cases there is no underlying skin abnormality although groin candidosis in men and women is more common in diabetics. Eczema or psoriasis affecting the skin flexures may be accompanied by secondary candidosis.

Candida infection with diaper dermatitis

Diaper rash in infants is a form of irritant eczema which is often secondarily infected with, among other organisms, *C. albicans*. The presence of yeasts may be suspected by the appearance of satellite pustules. This can be confirmed by culture.

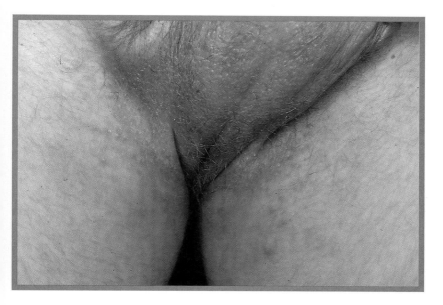

↑ **Fig. 81**
Candida intertrigo.

Interdigital candidosis

Infection of the finger or toe web spaces by *Candida* is more frequent in hot climates and it may be the commonest type of foot infection in military personnel in the tropics. Lesions are white with soggy-looking skin which is superficially eroded (**Fig. 82**). Between the toes, *Candida* may be a secondary invader in a lesion primarily caused by a dermatophyte.

Candidosis of the nails

Paronychia are acute or chonic infections of the nail folds caused by *C. albicans* or other *Candida* species such as *C. parapsilosis* (**Fig. 83**). They occur in patients who are likely to immerse their hands frequently in water or whose occupations involve cooking. They may also occur in patients with severe perniosis (chilblains). In addition to swelling of the nail fold, pain and intermittent discharge of pus, the lateral border of the nail may be undermined with onycholysis. Other causes of paronychia are staphylococcal and Gram-negative bacterial infections. The latter often coexist with *Candida*.

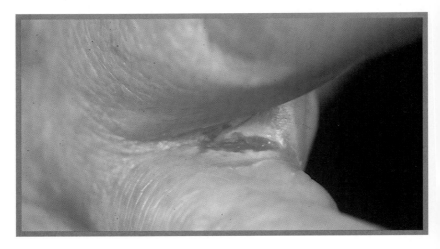

↑ Fig. 82
Interdigital candidosis.

Nail plate invasion due to *Candida* may occur in the presence of paronychia or in the syndrome of chronic mucocutaneous candidosis. In addition some patients may develop genuine nail plate invasion and destruction, particularly if there is underlying Raynaud's disease or Cushing's syndrome. Here the nail plate is seldom grossly thickened but onycholysis and terminal erosion both occur (**Fig. 84**).

→ Fig. 83
Paronychia due to
***Candida*.**

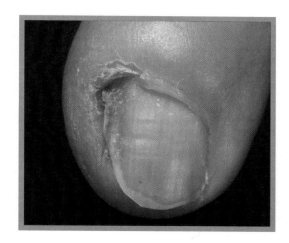

→ Fig. 84
Onychomycosis due
to *Candida*.

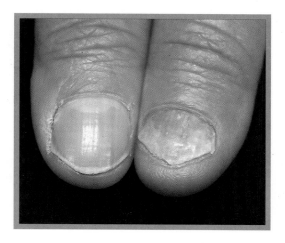

Other forms of *Candida* infection

Generalized cutaneous candidosis is a rare condition which is seen in newborn infants where the mother has a vaginal *Candida* infection prior to vaginal delivery. The baby's skin is covered with multiple pustules against a background of erythema.

Chronic mucocutaneous candidosis

The rare syndrome of chronic mucocutaneous candidosis (CMC) usually presents in childhood or infancy with oral, nail and cutaneous infection which recurs despite treatment. The classification of CMC is shown in **Figure 85**. Other chronic skin infections such as warts (papilloma viruses) and dermatophytosis may also be associated. An adult form also exists. The oral lesions are usually of the chronic pseudomembranous or plaque type. The skin may be covered with crusted plaques (the so-called *Candida* granuloma), particularly where the infection has spread to the face or scalp. The fingernail changes affect the nail plates, nail folds and periungual skin, all of which may be severely dystrophic (**Fig. 86**).

Classification of chronic mucocutaneous candidosis (CMC)

Childhood onset

Inherited CMC
       – autosomal recessive type
       – autosomal dominant type
CMC associated with polyendocrinopathy (usually hypoparathyroidism, hypoadrenalism)
Idiopathic CMC associated with hypothyroidism

Adult onset

CMC associated with thymoma
CMC associated with systemic lupus erythematosus

↑ **Fig. 85**
Classification of chronic mucocutaneous candidosis (CMC).

A large number of immunologic abnormalities have been thought to be associated with this condition, but with few exceptions these have altered over time and with therapy. For this reason it is likely that the real defect(s) in most patients with this condition remains unknown. The immunologic investigation of children with this abnormality is therefore not necessary unless they have very extensive lesions or a history suggestive of abnormal responses to other infections such as chicken pox or boils. Here it is worth excluding functional leukocyte abnormalities, such as chronic granulomatous disease, although affected patients usually have a history of internal infection. With the exception of bronchiectasis, most patients with CMC do not have internal disease, although the severely affected patient may later develop systemic infections such as tuberculosis.

Many patients with CMC develop a spontaneous remission as they get older, but some may deteriorate. As there is a wide range of clinical expression in this syndrome all patients should be followed up closely.

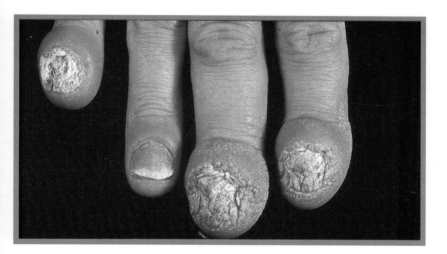

↑ **Fig. 86**
Chronic mucocutaneous candidosis.

Laboratory diagnosis

The presence of yeasts and filaments in a KOH preparation of skin or in a Gram-stained smear of exudate will confirm a *Candida* infection (**Figs 87&88**). Cultures on glucose–peptone agar or malt extract agar yield colonies after 24–48 hours' incubation at 37°C (**Fig. 89**). Their subsequent identification as *C. albicans* is made by demonstrating germ tubes after incubating the yeasts for 2–3 hours in serum, or by the formation of chlamydospores in a carbohydrate medium such as Rice/Tween agar (**Figs 90&91**).

Media are now available for primary isolation where *C. albicans* can be distinguished by developing a characteristic color. This technique gives an early identification of *C. albicans* and also an indication of the presence of mixed cultures. For further confirmation and for the identification of other yeast species biochemical tests must be performed. The assimilation pattern of individual carbohydrates can be determined using commercial systems.

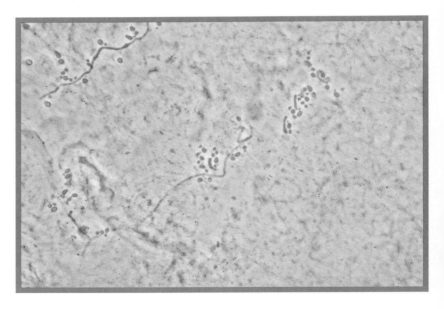

↑ **Fig. 87**
Skin in 30% KOH showing hyphae and yeasts.

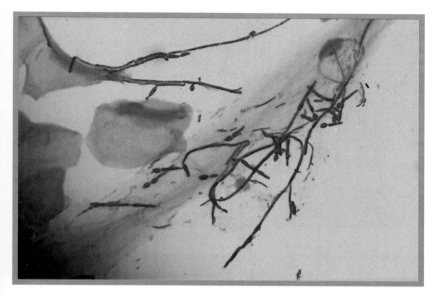

↑ **Fig. 88**
Vaginal exudate showing Gram-positive filaments and yeasts.

→ **Fig. 89**
Colonies of
Candida
***albicans* after**
48 hours'
incubation at
37°C.

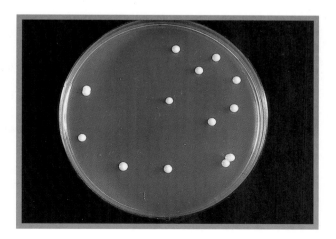

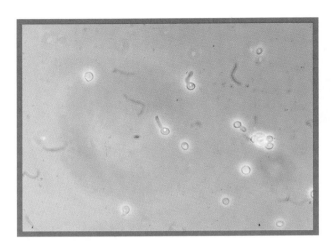

← **Fig. 90**
Germ tubes in serum after incubation of the yeasts for 2 hours at 37°C are diagnostic of *Candida albicans*.

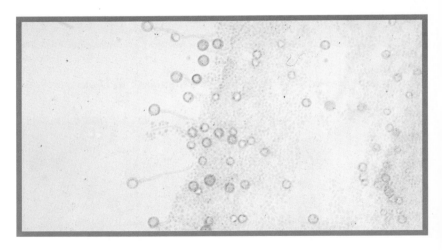

↑ **Fig. 91**
Identification of *Candida albicans* can also be made by the demonstration of chlamydospores at the tips of filaments after culturing on a Rice/Tween agar at 26°C for 48 hours.

The management of candidosis

Most superficial *Candida* infections respond to topical nystatin, azoles or amorolfine. In oral infections, nystatin lozenges or suspension, and amphotericin B lozenges are useful, at least for uncomplicated infections, although the taste of the medication is bitter. Miconazole oral gel is better tolerated by infants. When treating patients with oral candidosis associated with dentures, these should be removed overnight and cleaned with saline or a disinfectant before they are replaced. For infections in immunocompromised patients, it is often necessary to use an orally absorbed drug such as fluconazole, itraconazole or ketoconazole. In AIDS patients the doses of itraconazole (200mg) and ketoconazole (400mg) are double those used ordinarily, as absorption may be impaired due to achlorhydria. If possible, treatment is stopped in AIDS patients after achieving remission and then recurrences re-treated as necessary. Continuous therapy should be avoided.

For vaginal infections topically applied azoles, eg clotrimazole, sulconazole, econazole or miconazole, for a single vaginal dose are available usually in tablet form. Longer topical regimens can also be used. Where topical therapy is unacceptable, oral therapy with a single dose of fluconazole (150mg) or itraconazole (400mg) can be used. There is no magic answer to chronic or relapsing vaginal candidosis. In all cases it is important to confirm that the recurrence of symptoms really is accompanied by the presence of *Candida*. Longer-term therapy with a course of oral fluconazole or itraconazole over 2–3 weeks, followed by topical therapy with clotrimazole or even betadine once or twice weekly over 3 months, may occasionally bring a halt to repeated episodes of infection.

For paronychia, topical azoles are helpful if applied in solution form over 3–4 months or until the nail fold becomes less swollen. Similar results can be obtained with oral azoles such as itraconazole or ketoconazole. The latter drugs are the only effective therapies for genuine nail plate invasion due to *Candida*.

In the rare cases of chronic mucocutaneous candidosis, remission should be induced using fluconazole, itraconazole or ketoconazole. If possible, relapses should be treated when they occur by using intermittent azole therapy for 3–7 days if there is a severe clinical relapse. Resistance to ketoconazole has been described where the drug has been given continuously over several months in the face of continuing infection.

4.3 *Malassezia* infections

Malassezia yeasts (previously known as *Pityrosporum* or the lipophilic yeasts) are skin surface commensals which have also been associated with certain human diseases, the commonest of which are pityriasis versicolor, *Malassezia* (*Pityrosporum*) folliculitis and seborrheic dermatitis (including dandruff). In addition, these organisms cause infrequent systemic infections, usually in neonatal infants receiving intravenous lipid infusions.

Pityriasis versicolor

The pathogenesis of pityriasis versicolor is still poorly understood. The disease occurs in young adults and older individuals, less frequently in childhood. It is a common disease, particularly in the tropics in otherwise healthy subjects and there is no evidence of immunosuppression in these patients. However it has been associated with Cushing's syndrome and immunosuppressive therapy associated with transplantation, but not with AIDS. The pigmentary changes which characterize this infection are thought to follow the inhibition of melanin formation by substances, such as azaleic acid, produced by the

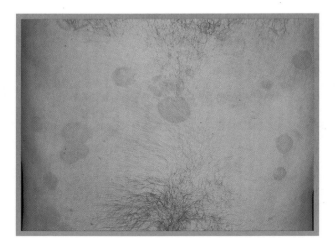

↑ Fig. 92
Pityriasis versicolor.

yeast in the epidermis.

The rash consists of multiple hypo- or hyperpigmented, occasionally red, macules which are distributed across the upper trunk (**Fig. 92**). With time these coalesce. The lesions are usually asymptomatic but show profuse fine scaling. Patients usually notice this infection because of its unsightly appearance. In the tropics, fear of other conditions such as leprosy may bring the patients to see a doctor.

Lesions can be highlighted by shining a Wood's light on the area. They fluoresce with a yellowish color, although this is generally a weak response and complete darkness as well as a powerful light source are necessary. Diagnosis is made by examination of skin scales in a mixture made up of equal parts of 30% KOH and Parker's permanent blue/black ink. The fungus quickly takes up the stain and consists of groups of thick-walled spherical yeasts together with angular hyphae in short lengths typical of the causative organism, *Malassezia furfur* (**Fig. 93**). Culture, which can be performed if lipid is included in the medium, is of no diagnostic value because the organism is also part of the normal human skin flora.

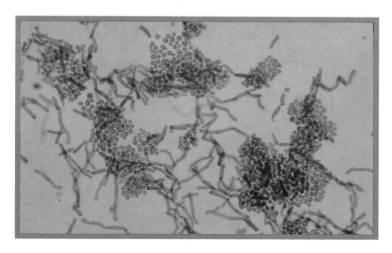

↑ **Fig. 93**
***Malassezia furfur* in skin stained with Parker's stain.**

Malassezia (Pityrosporum) folliculitis

A second condition associated with *Malassezia* yeasts is an itchy folliculitis on the back and upper trunk which often appears after a summer holiday and sun exposure (**Fig. 94**). *Malassezia* folliculitis is a clinically distinct condition most often seen in adolescents or young adult men. Lesions are itchy papules and pustules which are often widely scattered on the shoulders and back. The condition has to be distinguished from acne as it does not respond to the same range of treatments. A comparison of the features is given in **Figure 95**.

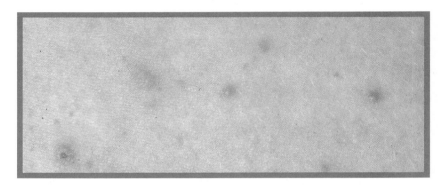

↑ **Fig. 94**
Malassezia **folliculitis.**

Malassezia/ (Pityrosporum) folliculitis and acne		
	***Malassezia* folliculitis**	**Acne vulgaris**
Comedones	No	Yes
Itch	Yes	Seldom
Facial lesions	Rare	Common
Precipitated by sun exposure	Common	Uncommon
Response to		
Antibiotics	No	Yes
Azoles	Yes	No

↑ **Fig. 95**
Malassezia **folliculitis and acne.**

Malassezia yeasts and seborrheic dermatitis.

The lipophilic yeasts are part of the normal skin flora and therefore any evidence that they are either directly or indirectly implicated in the pathogenesis of common skin diseases such as dandruff or seborrheic dermatitis is difficult to assess. However:

- *Malassezia* (*Pityrosporum*) yeasts may be found in large quantities in the scales of seborrheic dermatitis and dandruff;
- most patients with seborrheic dermatitis or dandruff respond to treatment with azole antifungal agents and this coincides with the disappearance of the yeasts;
- in animals it is possible to induce similar skin scaling by the application of *Malassezia* yeasts.

Seborrheic dermatitis is one of the earliest and most consistent conditions seen in patients with AIDS although it is also common in healthy individuals. The main clinical features of seborrheic dermatitis are the appearance of erythema together with greasy scales in the scalp, eyebrows and eyelashes, in the nasolabial folds, behind the ears and over the sternum (**Fig. 96**).

The relationship between infantile seborrheic dermatitis and these organisms is less well established although heavy colonization with *Malassezia* (*P. ovale*) has been documented in association with cradle cap eczema of the scalp.

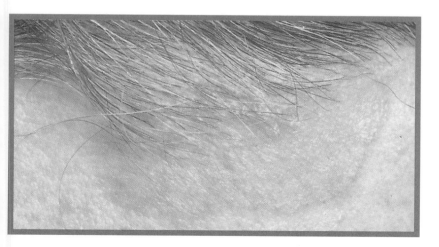

↑ Fig. 96
Seborrheic dermatitis.

Malassezia yeasts and facial eczema

Certain adult patients with erythema and eczema affecting the head and neck may respond to topical azole antifungals and also show immediate type hypersensitivity (prick tests) to extracts of *Malassezia*. Patients usually have a history of atopic disease, including eczema, or are atopic on family history. The condition is most often seen in young women.

Management of *Malassezia* infections

Pityriasis versicolor responds well to selenium sulfide used for at least 2 weeks, most topical azoles for 1–2 weeks, or oral ketoconazole 400mg as a single dose or itraconazole for 5 days of 200mg daily. Ketoconazole shampoo is also effective if given for 2–3 applications only. There are three potential problems in the management of this infection:

- relapse occurs very frequently, particularly in patients living in the tropics;
- skin discoloration take several months to disappear.

Patients often believe they are still infected after treatment because the skin color takes several months to revert to normal. They need to be reassured that this is normal and that they do not need more treatment.

Because of the persistence of the organism on the skin surface, in the early phases of therapy, direct microscopy of skin is a poor guide to the success of treatment.

Malassezia folliculitis is difficult to treat. Oral ketoconazole or ketoconazole shampoo are the most effective therapies although itraconazole is an alternative (7–10 days). Unfortunately, topical therapies seldom work well.

Seborrheic dermatitis. While conventional therapy with low- to medium-strength topical corticosteroids or tar-based preparations may be helpful, most patients with seborrheic dermatitis respond well to topical or oral azole therapy. The combination of an azole with hydrocortisone may be effective. Relapse is frequent whatever the therapy used.

4.4 *Scytalidium* infections

Scytalidium dimidiatum (formerly known as *Hendersonula toruloidea*), a plant pathogen found in the tropics and subtropics and *S. hyalinum*, which has so far been isolated only from man, cause infections of the skin which mimic the dry-type infections associated with *Trichophyton rubrum*. These conditions are seen frequently in endemic areas where the rate of infection may equal or even exceed that of the dermatophytes. They are found in Africa, the West Indies, the Indian subcontinent and the Far East as well as parts of the USA. In temperate countries, *Scytalidium* infections are mainly seen in immigrants from tropical regions.

The infection presents with scaling of the soles and palms (**Fig. 97**) and cracking between the toes. Nail dystrophy is common, often with dark discoloration of the nails, and onycholysis without significant thickening is frequently seen (**Fig. 98**); some patients have nail fold swelling. The clinical features of *S. dimidiatum* and *S. hyalinum* infections are indistinguishable. Lesions may often be asymptomatic. It is important to recognize these infections since they show no response to most antifungal drugs. A comparison of the features of *Scytalidium* infections and dermatophytosis is given in **Figure 99**.

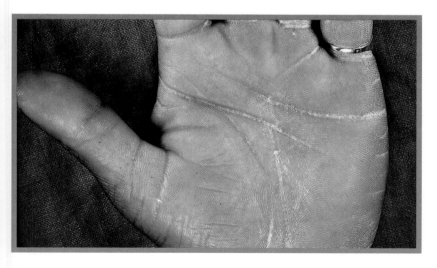

↑ **Fig. 97**
Scytalidium **infection of the hand.**

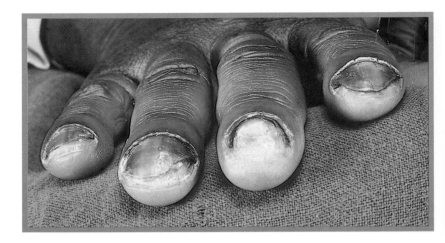

↑ **Fig. 98**
Nail infection due to *Scytalidium*.

***Scytalidium* infections and dermatophytosis**		
	Scytalidium	**Dermatophyte**
Site	Feet, hands	Feet, hands, body, groin
Itch	Sometimes	Usual
Prevalence	Origins tropics or subtropics	Worldwide
Nails	Little thickening	Thickened particularly on fingers

↑ **Fig. 99**
***Scytalidium* infections and dermatophytosis.**

The features seen on examination of infected skin in a KOH preparation can be recognized and identified as characteristic of a *Scytalidium* infection. The filaments are uneven in width and have a double-contoured appearance due to retraction of the cytoplasm from the hyphal cell wall (**Fig. 100**).

Both *Scytalidium* species are sensitive to cycloheximide, an agent commonly incorporated into mycologic media, therefore this antibiotic must be excluded if these fungi are to be isolated. Cultures of *S. dimidiatum* develop rapidly to form gray to black colonies which completely fill the Petri dish (**Fig. 101**). Some isolates grow more slowly. On microscopy there are chains of one- to two-celled arthroconidia which become dark brown in color (**Fig. 102**). *S. hyalinum* has white colonies (**Fig. 103**).

The management of *Scytalidium* infections is difficult. These infections do not respond to griseofulvin and insufficient evidence is available at present to know whether terbinafine, itraconazole or amorolfine will be useful clinically.

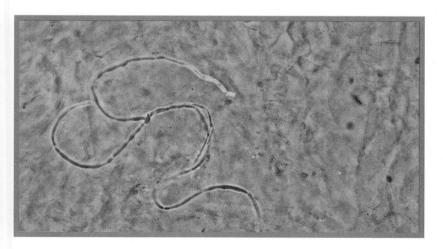

↑ **Fig. 100**
KOH preparation of skin infected with *Scytalidium*.

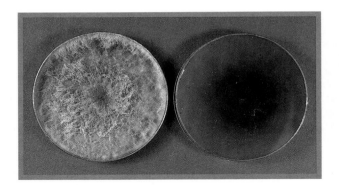

← Fig. 101
Scytalidium dimidiatum colony. (Courtesy of Dr M K Moore, St John's Institute of Dermatology, London)

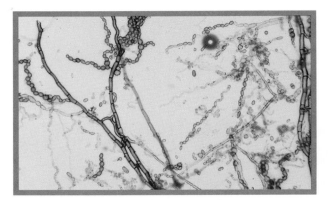

← Fig. 102
Microscopy of *Scytalidium dimidiatum* culture showing pigmented arthroconidia. (Courtesy of Dr M K Moore, St John's Institute of Dermatology, London)

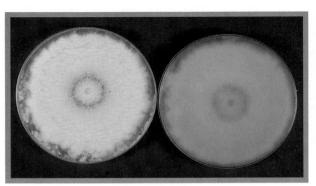

← Fig. 103
Colony of *Scytalidium hyalinum*. (Courtesy of Dr M K Moore, St John's Institute of Dermatology, London)

4.5 Onychomycosis

A variety of filamentous nondermatophyte organisms may cause nail infections, particularly as secondary invaders after damage by trauma or disease. Toenails, especially hallux nails, are affected more than fingernails and there are no associated skin lesions. Nails infected with *Scopulariopsis brevicaulis* develop a brown discoloration and a crumbly texture (**Fig. 104**). The appearance of the fungus in the KOH preparation may show features suggestive of a nondermatophyte infection such as the thick-walled conidia

→ Fig. 104
Nail infected with
Scopulariopsis
brevicaulis.

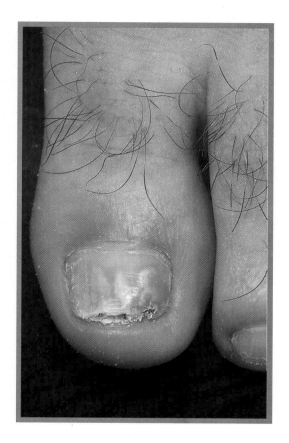

seen with *Scopulariopsis* (**Figs 105&106**) or the profuse branching of the hyphae to form fronds (see Fig. 110). As the fungi involved are common in the environment their significance in cultures of nail material must be interpreted with care. Several criteria must be considered, including the clinical appearance, history, features seen on microscopy, response to treatment and, if possible, repeated isolation of the same species.

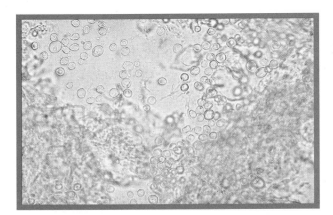

← Fig. 105 KOH preparation of a nail showing the thick-walled conidia typical of *Scopulariopsis* infection.

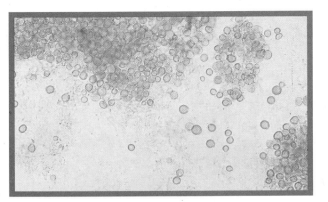

← Fig. 106 Nail infected with *Scopulariopsis* treated with Parker's stain. The conidia have taken up the blue color.

Cultures of nails suspected of a nondermatophyte infection should be made on a medium without cycloheximide. *Scopulariopsis brevicaulis* cultures have brown powdery colonies (**Fig. 107**) with conidia borne in chains on branched conidiophores (**Fig. 108**).

→ Fig. 107
Colony of
Scopulariopsis
brevicaulis.

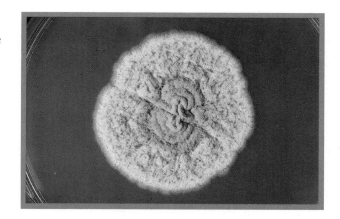

→ Fig. 108
Microscopy of
Scopulariopsis
brevicaulis
showing
chains of
rough-walled,
lemon-shaped
conidia borne
on branched
conidiophores.

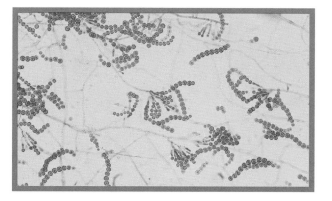

Other fungi may also be isolated from dystrophic nails. These include species of *Acremonium, Fusarium* and *Aspergillus*. A clinical appearance of superficial white onychomycsosis is characteristic of nails infected with nondermatophytes (**Fig. 109**). Microscopy shows profuse hyphae, branching to form fronds (**Fig. 110**). The colonies of *Acremonium strictum* are white to

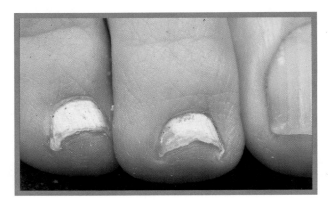

← **Fig. 109**
White crumbly patches on the surface of nails infected with *Acremonium* species.

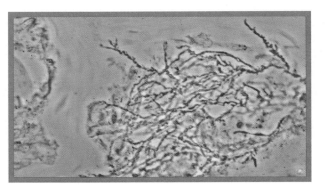

← **Fig. 110**
***Acremonium* species in a wet preparation of a nail showing characteristic fronds of the hyphae.**

pink, sticky in texture and become folded (**Fig. 111**). The conidia are formed at the tips of phialides, often remaining stuck together in balls (**Fig. 112**).

For the management of nondermatophyte nail infections, if only one nail is infected, topical application of a nail lacquer such as amorolfine or tioconazole could be used either alone or following removal of the nail.

→ Fig. 111 Colonies of *Acremonium strictum.*

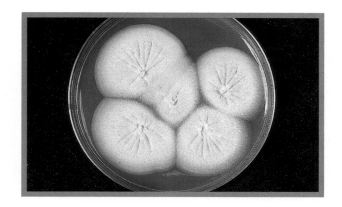

→ Fig. 112 Microscopy of *Acremonium strictum* showing conidia in clumps at the tips of tapering phialides.

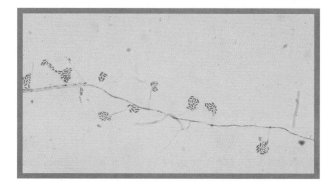

4.6 Other miscellaneous infections

White piedra

This is a chronic infection of the shafts of pubic, axillary or beard hairs. It may also affect the scalp. Irregular soft white nodules composed of hyphae and arthroconidia are formed around the hairs (**Fig. 113**). The nodules stain rapidly with Parker's stain (**Fig. 114**). The infection is caused by the *Trichosporon* species *T. inkin* (**Fig. 115**) or *T. cutaneum* which were previously included in the complex species *T. beigelii*.

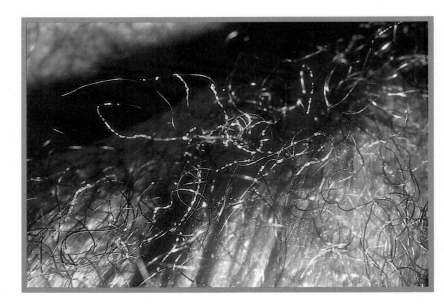

↑ **Fig. 113**
 White piedra. (Courtesy of the late Dr C Kalter, Walter Reed Army Medical Centre, USA)

→ Fig. 114
Pubic hairs in
Parker's stain
showing
nodules.

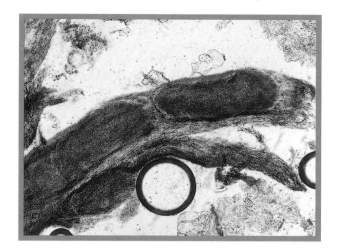

→ Fig. 115
Colonies of
*Trichosporon
inkin.*
(Courtesy of
Dr M K Moore,
St John's
Institute of
Dermatology,
London)

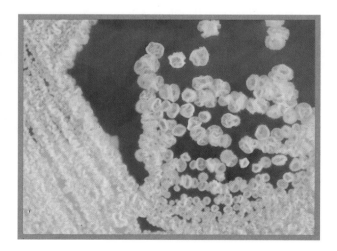

Black piedra

This is an infection of scalp hairs caused by *Piedraia hortae*. It is a rare infection confined to the tropics. The hairs have dense black nodules attached to the shaft which are variable in size and often visible to the naked eye (**Fig. 116**). When the nodules are crushed in KOH, asci containing fusiform ascospores may be seen (**Fig. 117**). Cultures produce dark brown or black colonies of *P. hortae* (**Fig. 118**).

For the management of both types of piedra, cutting or shaving off affected hairs is the simplest form of treatment. Topical application of an imidazole is effective.

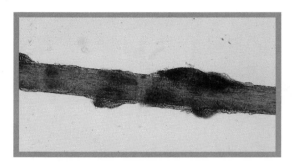

← Fig. 116
Black piedra hair.

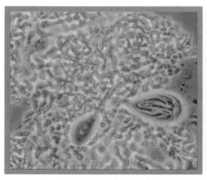

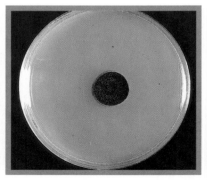

↑ Fig. 117
Nodule of black piedra in a wet preparation showing asci with ascospores. (Courtesy of Dr M K Moore, St John's Institute of Dermatology, London)

↑ Fig. 118
Colonies of *Piedraia hortae*.

Tinea nigra

This is an infection of palmar or plantar skin caused by a black yeast, *Phaeoannellomyces werneckii*. It is mainly seen in the tropics but can present in Europe and the USA. The main differential diagnosis is an acral melanoma as it presents as a flat pigmented mark on the hands or feet (**Fig. 119**). If the lesion is scraped with a scalpel it can be shown to be scaly. Lesions are usually solitary. When material is examined in KOH it shows branching septate pigmented hyphae (**Fig. 120**). The colonies of *P. werneckii* are pale and moist initially with blastoconidia but they become filamentous and dark-colored with age.

Suitable treatment is daily application of an imidazole or undecylenic acid which is continued for 2–3 weeks to avoid recurrence.

Fig. 119 →
Tinea nigra lesion.

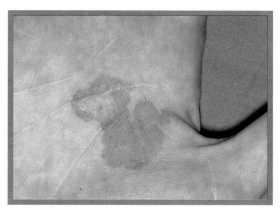

Fig. 120 →
Scales from tinea nigra in a KOH preparation.

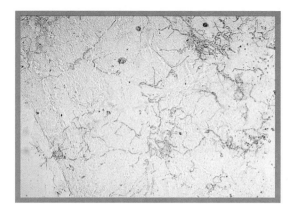

Otomycosis

This is a superficial, chronic or subacute infection of the outer ear canal characterized by inflammation, scaling, pruritis and pain. Fungi are often superimposed on a bacterial infection. Hyphae may be seen in exudate (**Fig. 121**). *Aspergillus* species, particularly *A. niger* (**Figs 122&123**), are involved as well as other fungi such as *Scedosporium* and *Candida* species. For treatment topical imidazoles are effective.

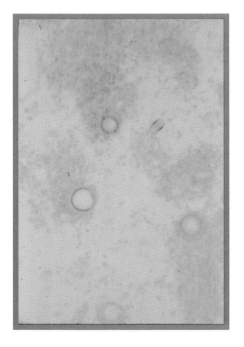

← **Fig. 121
Exudate from ear
discharge.**

→ Fig. 122
Culture of
black colonies
of *Aspergillus
niger.*

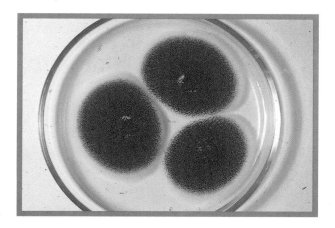

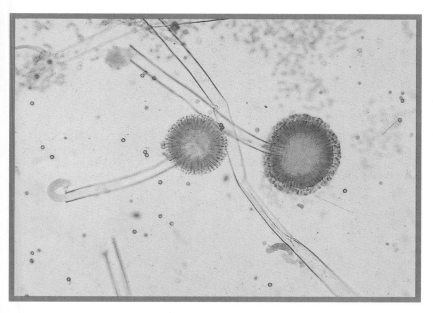

↑ Fig. 123
Microscopy of *Aspergillus niger.*

Mycotic keratitis

This is an infection of the corneal surface which usually follows an injury to the eye (**Fig. 124**). Hyphae may be demonstrated in scrapings taken from the cornea (**Fig. 125**). A wide range of fungi have been isolated from eye infections but *Aspergillus (A. fumigatus)*, *Fusarium (F. solani)* and *Candida* species are

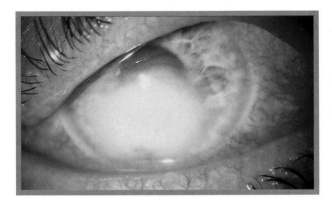

← **Fig. 124 Mycotic keratitis. (Courtesy of Mr T Gray, Bascom Palmer Eye Institute, Miami)**

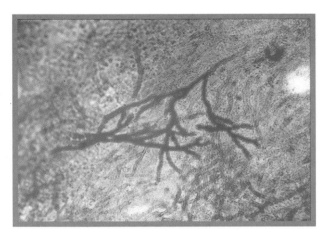

← **Fig. 125 Filaments in corneal scrapings.**

prominent among the pathogens. *Fusarium* species have pale colored colonies, pink, mauve or white (**Fig. 126**). The curved shape of the macroconidia is typical of the genus (**Fig. 127**).

The treatment of mycotic keratitis will be dependent on the causative species.

→ **Fig. 126**
Colony of *Fusarium solani*.

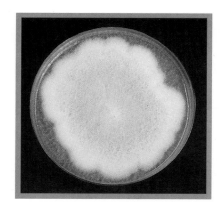

→ **Fig. 127**
Microscopy of *Fusarium solani* showing curved multicellular macroconidia.

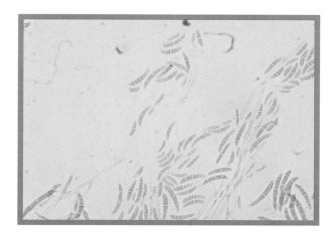

5 | Subcutaneous Mycoses

The subcutaneous mycoses are infections of implantation. In most cases they develop following traumatic injury and the inoculation of environmental organisms into the host where they affect the subcutaneous tissue, skin and other adjacent structures. These infections are mainly found in the tropics and subtropics; they are sporadic in occurrence and they chiefly affect manual workers. The most frequently encountered are:
- mycetoma,
- sporotrichosis,
- chromoblastomycosis
- phaeohyphomycosis.

Other rarer infections include lobomycosis and subcutaneous zygomycosis.

Most subcutaneous mycoses are chronic infections which may present years after a patient has left an endemic area. They should therefore be considered as potential causes of illness in immigrants from tropical countries. A definitive diagnosis of a subcutaneous infection can often be made by histopathology with subsequent culture of the pathogen for confirmation.

5.1 Mycetoma

Mycetoma (Madura foot) is a chronic infection caused by fungi (eumycetoma) or actinomycetes (actinomycetoma). The characteristic feature of this infection is the formation of large granules or grains within abscesses which drain through sinuses onto the skin. Extension of the infection can lead to involvement of the bones.

The condition is seen throughout a wide range of tropical countries from Mexico to the Far East but it occurs most frequently in dry regions such as Sudan and parts of India. The causative organisms are usually environmental saprophytes and plant parasites. Many of the fungal causes of eumycetoma are found in plant material; the actinomycetes are present in the soil. The infection may follow implantation of contaminated material such as a thorn, but this can occur months or even years before clinical presentation.

Clinical features

The main sites involved are feet, legs and hands but lesions on the chest and scalp have been reported. Patients initially present with a hard subcutaneous swelling; later, sinus tracts develop over the area. There is progressive swelling and deformity (**Fig. 128**). Pain is variable and there is usually localized sweating on the surface of the mycetoma. Small but visible grains are characteristically present in the discharge from the sinuses (**Fig. 129**) and these can be black, white, yellow or red in color. X-rays show lytic lesions in the bone with periosteal proliferation and erosion.

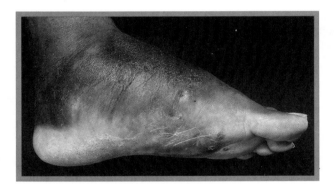

← **Fig. 128
Mycetoma of
the foot.**

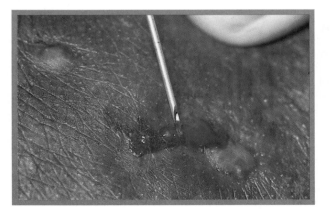

← **Fig. 129
Draining of a
sinus in a
mycetoma
opened with a
sterile needle,
showing the
grains.**

Laboratory diagnosis

A critical step in the diagnosis is to distinguish between fungal and actinomycete causes as the latter are treatable with chemotherapy and the former generally require surgery. Preliminary examination of a potassium hydroxide (KOH) preparation of exudate will reveal grains 50–500µm in diameter and the presence of pigment and hyphae is noted. Black grains are always due to fungi and red grains are caused by actinomycetes. White (or yellow) grains may be due to either group of organisms. The presence of hyphae 2–6µm wide indicates a eumycetoma but actinomycete filaments are ≤1µm across. The chief causative organisms of mycetoma are given in **Figure 130.**

Principal causes of mycetoma

Organism	Color of grain	Prevalence
Eumycetoma		
Madurella mycetomatis	Black	Africa, India, Middle East
M. grisea	Black	New World
Leptosphaeria senegalensis	Black	Africa
Scedosporium apiospermum	White/yellow	Worldwide
Fusarium species	White/yellow	Worldwide
Acremonium species	White/yellow	Worldwide
Actinomycetoma		
Actinomadura madurae	White/yellow	Africa, India
A. pelletieri	Red	Africa, India
Streptomyces somaliensis	White/yellow	Africa, India, Middle East
Nocardia brasiliensis	White/yellow	Central/South America
N. asteroides	White/yellow	Worldwide

↑ **Fig. 130**
Principal causes of mycetoma.

On histopathology, the characteristic appearance of the two types of grain is apparent with hematoxylin and eosin (H&E) staining. The fungal filaments in grains from eumycetoma are also easily demonstrated with periodic acid–Schiff (PAS) stain (**Fig. 131**). The fine filaments present in actinomycetoma give an amorphous appearance to the grain when viewed in section (**Fig. 132**).

Cultures may be prepared on glucose–peptone agar but a richer medium such as brain–heart infusion (BHI) agar (Difco) is often used. For the recovery of the organisms from eumycetoma, antibacterial antibiotics such as chloramphenicol (0.005%) or gentamicin (0.025%) may be included but cycloheximide should not be added. Incubation is at 26–28°C for 3–6 weeks.

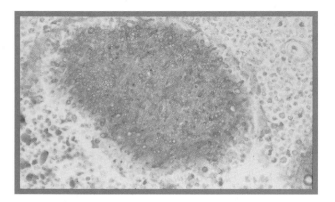

← **Fig. 131** **Section of a pale grain eumycetoma. Filaments are 2–6μm in width and are septate (PAS stain).**

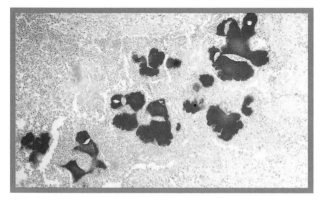

← **Fig. 132** **Section of an actino-mycetoma grain caused by** *Actinomadura pelletieri.* **The filaments are 1μm in width (H&E stain).**

A wide variety of fungi can cause this disease and identification by a specialist laboratory is recommended. **Figures 133&134** show an agent from a pale grain eumycetoma, *Scedosporium apiospermum*, and an isolate from a black grain, *Madurella mycetomatis*, is shown in **Figures 135&136**.

→ Fig. 133 *Scedosporium apiospermum*. The colonies are floccose, initially white but becoming gray in color.

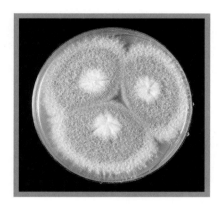

→ Fig. 134 Microscopic examination shows ovoid conidia produced singly at the tips of conidiophores.

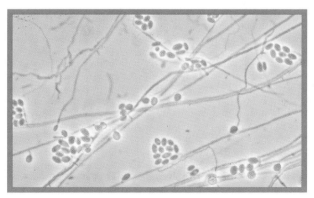

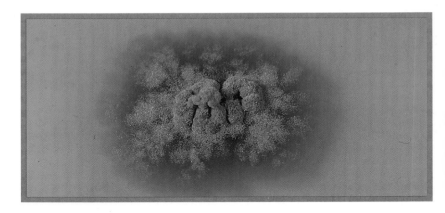

↑ Fig. 135
Madurella mycetomatis. A colony is slow growing and folded with a raised center. The color is gray to brown and a brown pigment diffuses into the medium.

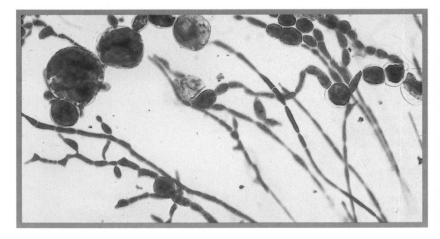

↑ Fig. 136
Microscopic examination shows septate hyphae, irregular in width with intercalary and terminal chlamydospores.

The actinomycetes responsible for actinomycetoma are isolated on media such as glucose–peptone agar, nutrient agar or blood agar in which all antibiotics are omitted. Incubation is at 30°C. The identification of the organisms relies on physiologic characteristics as well as morphology. Folded waxy colonies such as those shown in **Figures 137&138** are formed.

Management
The treatment of eumycetoma is difficult as responses to antifungal agents are unpredictable. However, ketoconazole and, to a lesser extent, itraconazole may be effective in patients with *Madurella mycetomatis* infections. Alternatives include griseofulvin, terbinafine or lipid-associated amphotericin B. In some cases surgery is necessary.The decision to operate should take into account current and future disability, and the availability of suitable prosthetic devices as some form of amputation is nearly always necessary.

Therapy for actinomycetoma ranges from sulfonamides and co-trimoxazole to dapsone. In addition, for the first 4–8 weeks a second drug such as rifampicin or streptomycin may be used. *Streptomyces somaliensis* infections are notoriously difficult to treat and other options such as fusidic acid or amikacin should be considered.

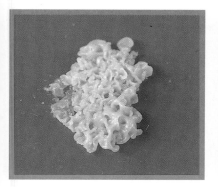

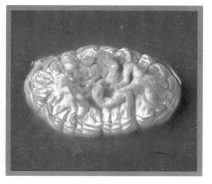

↑ **Fig. 137**
Actinomadura madurae. **Colony has a shiny, waxy, wrinkled surface and is white to yellow in color.**

↑ **Fig. 138**
Nocardia brasiliensis. **Colony is folded and raised with a chalky appearance on the surface. The color is white to orange.**

5.2 Sporotrichosis

Sporotrichosis is caused by the dimorphic fungus *Sporothrix schenckii* which is found in soil, on plant debris and on decaying vegetable material such as timber.

Infections occur over a wide geographic range in the tropics and subtropics including the southern USA, Japan and Australia but it has also been known in temperate climates. The disease is most prevalent, however, in central and northern South America and South Africa. It usually presents as a skin infection, cutaneous sporotrichosis, when the organism gains entry through traumatic injury, but systemic sporotrichosis featuring lung lesions or arthritis may also occur. Cutaneous sporotrichosis occurs sporadically. Certain occupational groups such as those who handle plant materials or soil (gardeners, florists, forestry workers) are frequently exposed to the organism and have been known to become infected. Miners have also acquired the disease from handling contaminated timber.

Clinical features
The clinical lesions are of two types, fixed and lymphangitic. Fixed lesions are solitary granulomas which ulcerate and are often confined to the face or exposed areas (**Fig. 139**). Satellite lesions may develop around the margin. They mostly resemble cutaneous leishmaniasis.

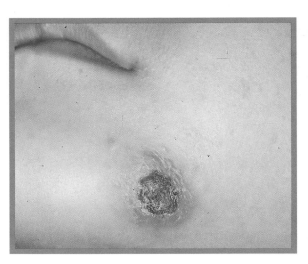

← **Fig. 139 Fixed lesion of sporotrichosis. (Courtesy of Dr F Montero-Gei, University of Costa Rica)**

Lymphangitic lesions commence with a primary granuloma or ulcer at the site of injury with secondary nodules appearing along the course of the draining lymphatics (**Fig. 140**). These resemble either *Mycobacterium marinum* infections (fish tank granuloma) or leishmaniasis. The nodules may ulcerate. Atypical presentations include plaques, chronic ulcers and mycetoma-like lesions.

Laboratory diagnosis
Histopathologic examination of a skin biopsy reveals few organisms. H&E staining may show isolated oval yeast cells surrounded by an eosinophilic substance which forms an asteroid body (**Fig. 141**).

→ Fig. 140 Lymphangitic lesions of sporotrichosis.

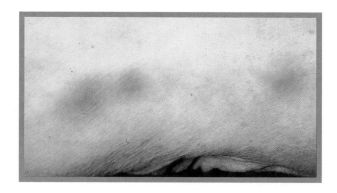

→ Fig. 141 Section of sporotrichosis. Asteroid body (stellate rays of eosinophilic material surrounding the location of a fungal cell. H&E).

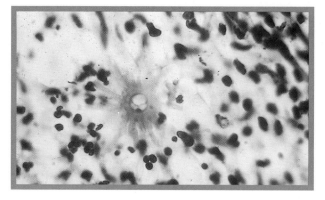

Culture is necessary to confirm the diagnosis, and colonies of *Sporothrix schenckii* are easily obtained. Material such as exudate from ulcers or a biopsy inoculated onto glucose–peptone agar or BHI agar, which may include both cycloheximide and chloramphenicol, will yield white or gray colonies at 26°C which become darker, sometimes black, as the culture matures. The colonies have a wrinkled surface and a moist texture (**Fig. 142**). On microscopy there are clusters of oval conidia, formed at the tips of the conidiophores in a palmate pattern (**Fig. 143**). Further confirmation of the identification is

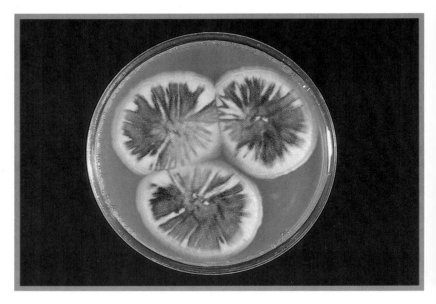

↑ **Fig. 142**
Colonies of *Sporothrix schenckii* isolated at 26°C.

obtained by subculturing isolates onto BHI agar and incubating at 37°C in order to convert the fungus to the yeast phase. Moist cream-colored colonies consisting of elongated yeasts develop under these conditions (**Fig. 144**).

Management
The classical treatment for sporotrichosis is a saturated solution of potassium iodide, from 1ml tid, when the dose is increased daily to 4–6ml tid to prevent intolerance . Alternatives include itraconazole or terbinafine.

→ Fig. 143 Microscopy of *Sporothrix schenckii* when grown at 26°C, showing conidia in a palmate arrangement on slender conidiophores.

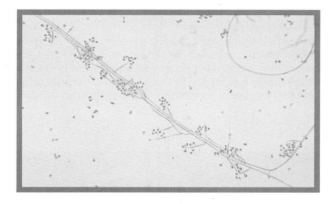

→ Fig. 144 Yeasts of *Sporothrix schenckii* developing at 37°C.

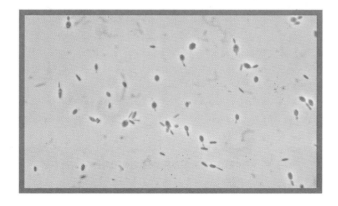

5.3 Chromoblastomycosis

Chromoblastomycosis is a chronic fungal infection affecting the dermis and epidermis with characteristic verrucous lesions on exposed sites such as the feet or the legs. The causative organisms are pigmented, or dematiaceous, fungi and the characteristic feature is the presence of pigmented fungal cells, in skin scrapings or biopsy material.

The infection occurs sporadically and rarely in the humid parts of the world. Its distribution covers Central and South America, Africa, particularly the Natal province in South Africa, Madagascar and the Far East including Japan. Those affected are usually agricultural workers and infection is assumed to follow implantation of environmental organisms which grow on plant debris.

Clinical features
The earliest skin lesion is a small papule slowly enlarging to form a verrucous, hyperkeratotic mass which can be up to 3cm in thickness (**Fig. 145**). These lesions may proliferate and spread on exposed sites such as the legs or hands. Occasionally lesions are flat and atrophic. Complications include secondary bacterial infection, lymphedema and squamous cell carcinoma.

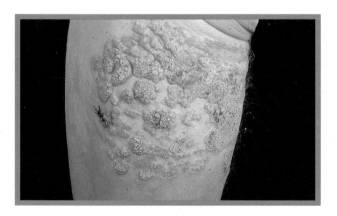

↑ **Fig. 145 Chromoblastomycosis lesions on the thigh.**

Laboratory diagnosis

Microscopy of KOH preparations of skin scrapings from the surface of lesions or of biopsy sections will show pigmented thick-walled muriform cells in the skin scales or deeper tissue. These pigmented cells can be seen in dermal granulomas, giant cells or the epidermis on histopathology. They may be single or in multiple-celled clusters which are produced after cell division by cross-wall formation and not by budding (**Fig. 146**).

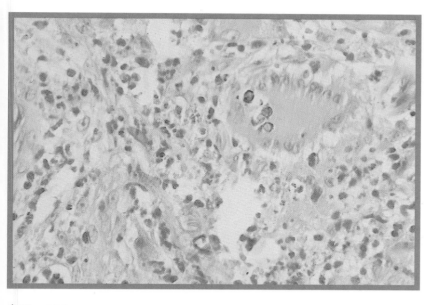

↑ Fig. 146
Section of chromoblastomycosis showing spherical, thick-walled brown fungal cells within a giant cell. The fungal cells are 5–12μm in diameter and may be septate (H&E).

Cultures of biopsy material, cut into small fragments, are made on glucose–peptone agar or BHI agar which may include both cycloheximide and chloramphenicol. Incubation is at 26–28°C for up to 6 weeks. The agents are all slow-growing, dematiaceous fungi which form very similar dark velvety colonies (**Fig 147**). The most frequent species are *Fonsecaea pedrosoi* and *Cladosporium carrionii.* Less common pathogens are *F. compacta, Phialophora verrucosa* and *Rhinocladiella aquaspersa.* Identification is largely made by studying the shape and mode of formation of the conidia (**Figs 148&149**) and confirmation of the species would be left to a specialist laboratory.

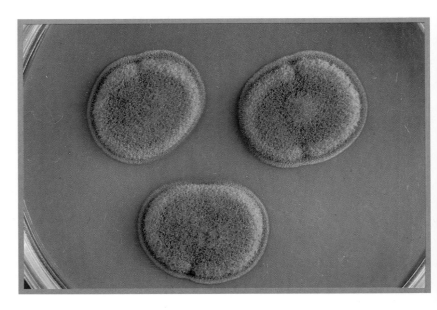

↑ **Fig. 147**
Colonies of *Fonsecaea pedrosoi.*

Management

Itraconazole with or without flucytosine is often successful. Terbinafine or flucytosine combined with amphotericin B may also be effective but flucytosine used alone may lead to resistance. Other alternatives include thiabendazole or the local application of heat. Surgery is not advised as it can lead to spread of the infection.

→ **Fig. 148 Microscopy of *Fonsecaea pedrosoi* showing chains of conidia.**

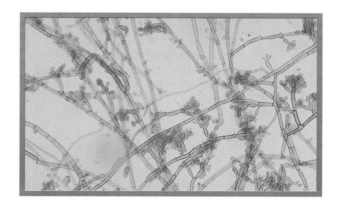

→ **Fig. 149 Microscopy of *Phialophora verrucosa* showing conidia formed in flask-shaped phialides.**

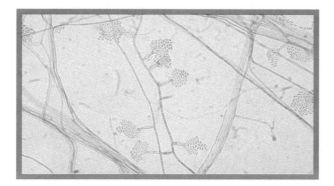

5.4 Phaeohyphomycosis

Localized subcutaneous infections forming granulomas, cysts or abscesses caused by a range of dematiaceous fungi come under the heading of pheohyphomycosis. These cases are rare and probably originate by implantation during an injury. They may occur in temperate as well as tropical areas. Also included in this group would be cutaneous alternariosis where the fungus, *Alternaria alternata* causes a form of granuloma in the cutaneous tissues.

Clinical features
The infections start with a tender nodule which may develop into a large cyst with no thickening of the overlying epidermis. The differential clinical diagnosis includes sebaceous and Baker's cysts.

Diagnosis
These infections are generally diagnosed after surgical excision when histopathology reveals the presence of pigmented septate hyphae in an inflammatory abscess wall (**Fig. 150**). The causative fungi vary in the degree of pigmentation formed *in vivo*, and it may be necessary to use a special stain, Fontana–Masson, to demonstrate the pigment in the fungal cells.

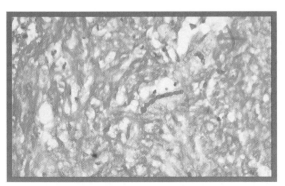

← **Fig. 150
Section of
phaeohyphomycosis
showing septate
hyphae (PAS).**

Cultures of fragments of biopsy tissue yield dark-colored fungi on glucose–peptone agar without cycloheximide. Most of the etiologic agents grow best at 30°C. An increasing number of fungi are known to cause phaeohyphomycosis, among them *Exophiala* species and *Bipolaris* species (**Figs 151&152**). Identification of these fungi should be left to a specialist laboratory.

Management
The usual treatment for this disease is excision together with an antifungal agent such as itraconazole.

→ **Fig. 151**
Dark colonies of *Bipolaris* species.

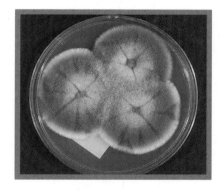

→ **Fig. 152**
Microscopy of *Bipolaris* species showing multicellular conidia with dark brown walls.

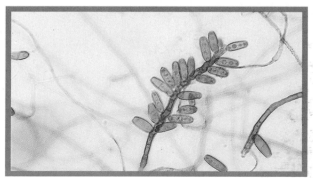

5.5 Other subcutaneous infections

Lobomycosis

This is a rare infection seen in Central and South America which resembles an inflammatory keloid scar. The organisms are present in tissue sections as chains of cells joined by a narrow tubular structure (**Fig. 153**). The fungus has never been isolated *in vitro* and its source is unknown. Treatment is surgical excision.

Zygomycosis

There are two forms of subcutaneous zygomycosis. These are found in Africa and Latin America. Infections due to *Conidiobolus coronatus* affect the central region of the face and the nose (**Fig. 154**) whereas those due to *Basidiobolus ranarum* usually involve a limb, the shoulder (**Fig. 155**) or pelvic area. Both present with painless but hard swellings which are usually well delineated. The fungi can be seen in biopsies as large aseptate hyphal fragments often surrounded by giant cells and eosinophils (**Fig. 156**).

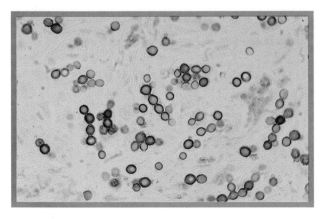

← **Fig. 153 Section of lobomycosis with a chain of cells (GMS).**

→ Fig. 154
Subcutaneous
zygomycosis of
the face.

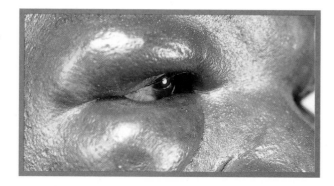

→ Fig. 155
Subcutaneous
zygomycosis of
the shoulder.
(Courtesy of
Prof E Drouhet,
Institut Pasteur,
Paris)

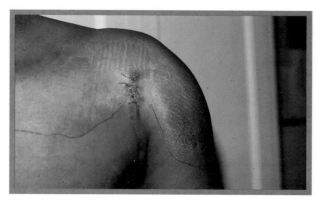

→ Fig. 156
Section showing
subcutaneous
zygomycosis.
Wide hyphae are
surrounded by
eosinophilic
material (H&E).

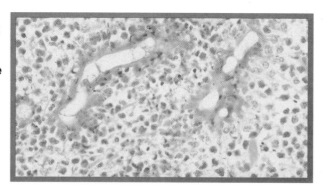

The cultures of *C. coronatus* and *B. ranarum* grow on media without cycloheximide (**Figs 157–161**).

Management
Treatment for these conditions is potassium iodide or itraconazole.

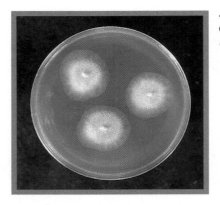

← Fig. 157
Colonies of *Conidiobolus coronatus*.

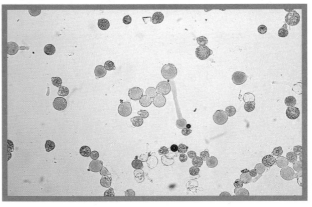

← Fig. 158
Conidia of *Conidiobolus coronatus* which are actively discharged from the tips of the conidiophores.

→ Fig. 159
Gray to tan colored, glabrous
and folded colony of
Basidiobolus ranarum.

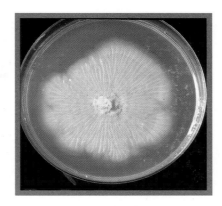

→ Fig. 160
Sporangia of
Basidiobolus
***ranarum* formed**
at the tip of
sporangiophore
from which they
are actively
discharged by a
projectile
mechanism.

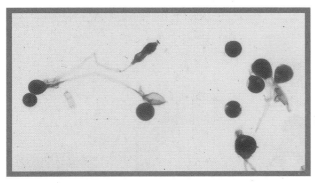

→ Fig. 161
Spherical, thick-
walled
zygospores of
Basidiobolus
***ranarum* formed**
after hyphal
fusion.

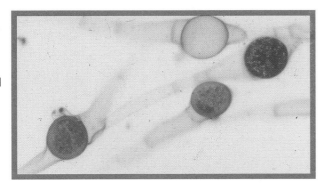

Diagnosis in color
Medical Mycology

6 Systemic Mycoses

The systemic mycoses are infections which predominantly affect internal systems or organs, such as the lungs or blood. There are two main groups of fungi which cause systemic disease: the primary respiratory pathogens and the systemic opportunistic fungal pathogens.
The endemic respiratory pathogens include:
- *Histoplasma capsulatum* var. *capsulatum* (histoplasmosis)
- *Histoplasma capsulatum* var. *duboisii* (African histoplasmosis)
- *Coccidioides immitis* (coccidioidomycosis)
- *Blastomyces dermatitidis* (blastomycosis)
- *Paracoccidioides brasiliensis* (paracoccidioidomycosis)
- *Penicillium marneffei*

Each mycosis has a definable endemic area.
The usual route of infection is through inhalation and there is a common pattern of illness associated with these infections (**Fig. 162**). Differences in clinical presentation reflect exposure to the pathogen (such as the inhalation of a large infective dose) and susceptibility of the individual. Patients with underlying immunologic defects such as HIV infection usually develop widespread disseminated disease.
The appropriate containment conditions should be utilized when handling pathologic material and cultures from any of the above diseases, as they all present a hazard to laboratory staff.

The systemic opportunistic fungal pathogens differ from the endemic mycoses in that they have a worldwide distribution. They may infect via various routes from the lungs to the gastrointestinal tract and they invade only in the presence of some underlying predisposition. The main infections are caused by:
- *Candida* species (systemic candidosis),
- *Aspergillus* species (aspergillosis),
- *Cryptococcus neoformans* (cryptococcosis),
- *Absidia, Rhizopus, Rhizomucor* species (zygomycosis)
- rarer systemic mycoses including infections due to *Fusarium* species, *Trichosporon* species and *Scedosporium apiospermum*.

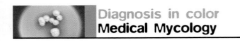

Cryptococcosis has some features of both the endemic respiratory and the opportunistic mycoses. In AIDS patients *Cryptococcus neoformans* is the most prevalent systemic fungal pathogen with infections occurring in 3–20% of that population.

Common pattern of disease caused by respiratory fungal pathogens

Form	Main site of infection	Symptoms/signs
Asymptomatic	Lung	Nil; positive DTH to antigen
Pulmonary		
Acute	Lung	Cough, fever, arthralgia, skin rashes
Chronic	Lung	Solitary/multiple defined granulomas. Cavitation or consolidation
Disseminated		
Acute	Widespread	Fever, weight loss, hepatosplenomegaly
Chronic	Focal involvement, eg adrenal, mouth, skin	Appropriate signs, eg Addison's disease, ulcers
Primary cutaneous	Skin	Local granuloma and peripheral lymphadenopathy

DTH = Delayed type hypersensitivity.

↑ Fig. 162
Common pattern of disease caused by respiratory fungal pathogens.

6.1 Endemic respiratory mycoses

Histoplasmosis

The classical or small form of histoplasmosis is endemic in many parts of the world, although not in Europe. It is mainly confined to the central and eastern USA, Central and South America, Africa and the Far East. Clinical disease follows the inhalation of conidia of the fungus, *Histoplasma capsulatum* var. *capsulatum,* which is a dimorphic fungus, found in soil contaminated with bird or bat excreta.

Clinical features

Asymptomatic infection occurs in endemic areas. Histoplasmin skin test surveys have revealed positive reactions in healthy individuals indicating exposure to the organism of over 80% of the population in parts of Kentucky and Tennessee in the USA and 60% in Trinidad to 20% or less in most African countries.

Acute pulmonary disease usually follows exposure to a source containing many organisms, such as bat-infested caves or chicken sheds. Symptoms include cough, fever, chest pain, arthralgia and erythema multiforme. Chest X-rays show a widespread mottling; fine calcification may develop later.

With chronic pulmonary infection there are asymptomatic nodules and cavitation. X-rays show apical shadows with cavities.

With acute disseminated histoplasmosis there is enlargement of the liver and/or spleen, bone marrow infiltration and purpura. Chest X-rays may show miliary mottling. In AIDS patients the main pattern of infection is this acute disseminated form together with fungemia and skin papules.

Chronic disseminated infection is characterized by ulcers or granulomas on the mouth, larynx and adrenals.

Laboratory diagnosis

Microscopy of body fluids and tissue biopsy reveals organisms which are very small and difficult to see. Special fungal stains such as Giemsa or periodic acid–Schiff (PAS) can be used on blood films or bone marrow. Histopathology of sections show small (2–4μm) oval to round yeasts which are intracellular (**Fig. 163**).

Cultures should be prepared at both 26°C and at 37°C in screw-capped bottles or tubes. The fungus grows in the mycelial phase at room temperature and in the yeast phase at 37°C where the preferred medium would be brain–heart infusion (BHI) agar. The mycelial phase produces white floccose colonies (**Fig. 164**) with large spherical rough-walled macroconidia (**Fig. 165**). Small microconidia are also present. The confirmation of identity of a mycelial isolate should also be obtained by converting from mycelial to the yeast phase after subculturing at 37°C using BHI agar (**Fig. 166**). Identification may also be made using an exoantigen test. This is an immunodiffusion assay for specific secreted antigen which is extracted from the fungal culture and reacted with a specific antibody. However, these techniques are being superseded by molecular methods.

For serologic diagnosis complement fixation tests (CFT) and immunodiffusion tests (ID) are available from specialists. Radioimmunoassay (RIA) for antigen detection, particularly in AIDS patients, is available.

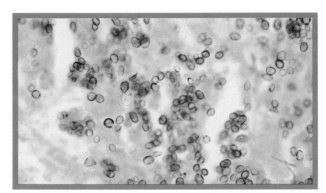

**← Fig. 163
Section of histoplasmosis showing small yeast cells (GMS).**

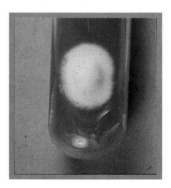

**↑ Fig. 164
Colony of *Histoplasma capsulatum* var. *capsulatum* at 26°C.**

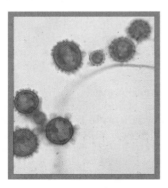

**↑ Fig. 165
Microscopy of *Histoplasma capsulatum* var. *capsulatum* showing large rough-walled macroconidia.**

Management

Intravenous amphotericin B is used for severely ill patients. Otherwise itraconazole is used and can also be given as maintenance therapy after remission.

African histoplasmosis is a related infection caused by *Histoplasma capsulatum* var. *duboisii*. It is confined to the central regions of Africa and can be distinguished from the classical form by:
- skin or bone lesions – lymphadenopathy are common;
- respiratory signs and symptoms – rare;
- serology – often negative; and
- histology – shows large oval to pear-shaped yeasts (6–10μm) in giant cells (**Fig. 167**).

Cultures are identical to classical histoplasmosis.

Treatment of *H. capsulatum* var. *duboisii* is with itraconazole.

**→ Fig. 166
Yeast phase of
*Histoplasma
capsulatum* var.
capsulatum at
37°C.**

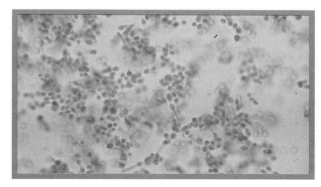

**→ Fig. 167
Section of
*Histoplasma
capsulatum* var.
duboisii
infection (PAS).**

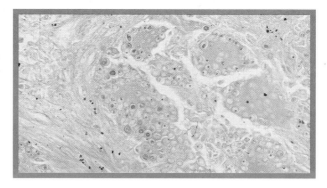

Coccidioidomycosis

Coccidioidomycosis is caused by the inhalation of spores of *Coccidioides immitis*, a soil-borne fungus which is found in the semidesert regions of North, Central and South America. Contamination of the atmosphere can increase heavily during dust storms leading to a surge in new cases of the disease. Disseminated infections may be found in healthy individuals, although they are more likely in immunocompromised subjects and diabetics. They are also commoner in women than men and in patients from certain ethnic groups such as Philipinos, Afro-Caribbeans and native Americans.

Clinical features

Asymptomatic infection is estimated to occur in up to 60% of the population in endemic areas of the USA, based on surveys using a coccidioidin skin test.

Symptoms of acute pulmonary infection include cough, fever and pleuritic pain. Spontaneous resolution occurs particularly when accompanied by erythema nodosum or erythema multiforme. Chest X-rays show focal consolidation, hilar lymphadenopathy and pleural effusion.

With chronic pulmonary infection there are asymptomatic pulmonary nodules or a chronic cough, with thin-walled lung cavities on X-ray.

Acute disseminated disease is a widespread infection with liver/spleen, lung, adrenal and skin involvement. This may occur in apparently healthy individuals as well as in immunosuppressed patients.

Chronic disseminated infection features a focal infection such as a meningitis or involvement of the skin or a single joint.

Laboratory diagnosis

Microscopy of sputum or material from abscesses or lung biopsy shows large spherules containing endospores that are visible in a wet mount. Histopathology of tissue prepared with fungal stains shows the morphology clearly of spherules in different stages of evolution in granulomatous stroma (**Fig. 168**).

Cultures of infected material on glucose–peptone agar or BHI agar yield colonies of *Coccidioides immitis* at 37°C (**Fig. 169**). The fungus is a white floccose mold which bears abundant arthroconidia formed by the regular septation of the hyphae. The viable arthroconidia alternate with smaller empty cells to give a characteristic appearance (**Fig. 170**). These conidia are highly infectious.

For serologic diagnosis CFT and ID tests are available.

Management

No treatment is necessary for the acute respiratory phase. Amphotericin B, itraconazole or fluconazole can be given for other forms of the disease. Treatment results are unpredictable, particularly for widely disseminated disease, meningitis and arthritis.

→ **Fig. 168**
Coccidioido-
mycosis of the
lung. Section
showing
spherules with
endospores
(PAS).

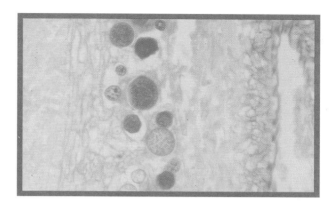

→ **Fig. 169**
Colony of *Coccidioides immitis*.

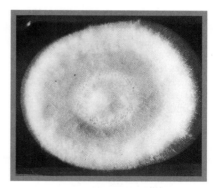

→ **Fig. 170**
Microscopic
appearance of
Coccidioides
immitis
showing the
typical
arthroconidia.

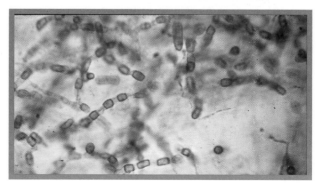

Blastomycosis

This infection is caused by the dimorphic fungus *Blastomyces dermatitidis*. It is found in the USA, Canada and North and Central Africa and is rare elsewhere. The environmental source of the fungus is unknown but is thought to be a habitat which is liable to flooding.

Clinical features

Asymptomatic infections probably occur but there is no commercial skin test antigen to determine the prevalence of blastomycosis in the population.

Acute pulmonary infection is rare and is mainly seen in children. The usual signs are cough, fever and dyspnoea.

Chronic pulmonary infection may coexist with disseminated extrapulmonary lesions. The symptoms include cough, fever and weight loss. Large pulmonary infiltrates or cavitation are seen on X-ray.

Acute disseminated disease is uncommon. Blastomycosis is rare in AIDS patients.

Chronic disseminated infection shows large skin plaques or abscesses, bone lesions and abscesses of the epididymis, often together with lung lesions.

Laboratory diagnosis

Microscopy of sputum, pus or tissue in KOH mounts shows large yeasts, 8–10μm, with buds forming on a broad base. These are seen clearly when stained in histopathologic sections (**Fig. 171**).

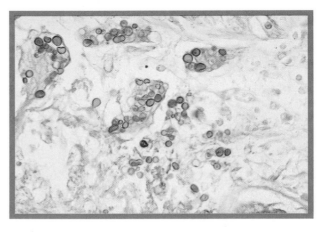

← **Fig. 171 Section of brain tissue infected with blastomycosis showing large, thick-walled yeasts which have a broad base to the bud (PAS).**

Cultures need to be made at 26°C and 37°C as the species is dimorphic. The mycelial phase grows at 26°C on primary isolation. The colonies are white to tan-colored and floccose (**Fig. 172**), which on microscopy show smooth-walled oval conidia borne singly on the sides of the hyphae (**Fig. 173**). Conversion to the yeast phase (**Fig. 174**) is achieved by placing subcultures at 37°C on enriched media such as BHI agar.

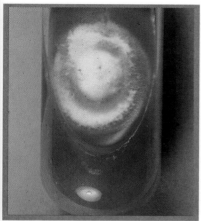

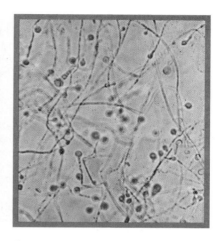

↑ **Fig. 172**
Colony of *Blastomyces dermatitidis* at 26°C.

↑ **Fig. 173**
Microscopy of *Blastomyces dermatitidis* showing oval conidia.

→ **Fig. 174**
Yeasts of *Blastomyces dermatitidis* grown at 37°C.

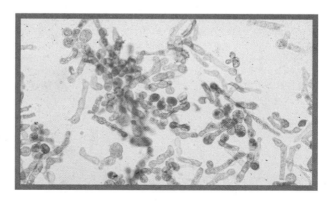

Serology is positive using ID but cross reactions occur with the other dimorphic pathogens.

Management
Itraconazole is the most effective treatment but alternatives include amphotericin B and ketoconazole.

Paracoccidioidomycosis

This infection is caused by the dimorphic fungus *Paracoccidioides brasiliensis,* which occurs throughout Central and South America except for Chile. The habitat of the pathogen is unknown. Although exposure rates are assumed to be similar in both men and women, the disease is 40 times more common in men.

Clinical features

Asymptomatic infections are estimated to occur in up to 30% of healthy individuals in endemic areas on the evidence of positive intradermal skin tests.

Acute pulmonary infection is unknown.

Chronic pulmonary infection is a common manifestation of the disease, with large opacities seen on chest X-ray. Symptoms include cough, fever and weight loss.

Chronic disseminated disease affects the larynx, lymph nodes and mucocutaneous regions such as the mouth, eyes and anus, where there may be ulceration.

A childhood disseminated form of paracoccidioidomycosis is a widespread infection affecting numerous sites and is difficult to treat.

Paracoccidioidomycosis is not common in AIDS patients.

Laboratory diagnosis

Wet preparations of exudate smears and sputum show large multiple budding yeast cells where the buds are arranged around the parent cell like a ship's wheel. A similar appearance is seen on histopathology (**Fig. 175**).

Cultures on glucose–peptone agar or BHI agar incubated at 26°C and 37°C show the dimorphic nature of the pathogen. A mycelial form grows at 26°C and a yeast phase at 37°C on enriched medium (**Fig. 176**).

For serologic diagnosis ID and CFT are used.

Management

Itraconazole is the most effective drug. Alternatives include amphotericin B and ketoconazole.

→ **Fig. 175 Section showing multiple budding yeasts in paracoccidioidomycosis (GMS).**

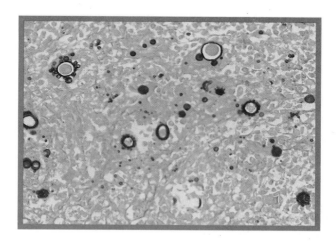

→ **Fig. 176 Yeasts showing multiple budding grown at 37°C.**

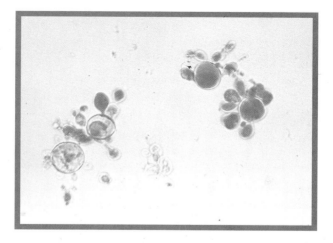

Penicillium marneffei infection

Penicillium marneffei is a mycelial fungus which causes disease in Southeast Asia, particularly Thailand and China. It causes infections in both healthy and immunosuppressed individuals, including AIDS patients. Its habitat is unknown, but naturally occurring infections have been found in bamboo rats.

Clinical features

Asymptomatic infection has not been proven.

With subacute or chronic pulmonary infection the clinical features range from a single lesion to miliary spread.

Disseminated infection may affect liver, spleen, bone marrow and skin. Over 50% of patients have skin lesions; this is the form seen in AIDS patients.

Laboratory diagnosis

Microscopy of tissue shows small organisms, 2–5µm. Giemsa stains may help visualize fungi in macrophages. On histopathology these small ovoid or curved organisms can be seen dividing by transverse fission following the formation of septa (**Fig. 177**).

Cultures on glucose–peptone agar or BHI agar at 26°C yield colonies of *P. marneffei* which have a gray surface and a red pigment diffusing into the medium

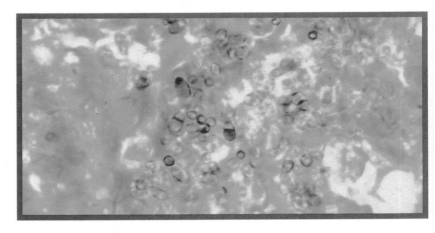

↑ **Fig. 177**
Section showing infection with *Penicillium marneffei*. Small fungal cells show septation (GMS).

(Fig. 178). The microscopic features are sporing heads typical of the *Penicillium* genus with conidia being borne in chains on a branched conidiophore **(Fig. 179)**.

For serologic diagnosis there are no commercial tests available. However, this fungus cross reacts in some serodiagnostic tests for *Aspergillus*.

Management
Treatment of severe cases requires amphotericin B, but otherwise itraconazole daily is effective. This should be given to AIDS patients for long-term suppression of relapse.

→ **Fig. 178**
Colony of *Penicillium marneffei*. (Courtesy of Dr D W Warnock, PHLS Mycology Reference Laboratory, Bristol)

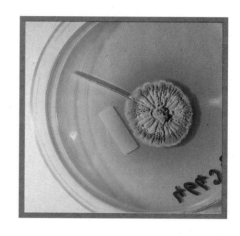

→ **Fig. 179 Microscopy of *Penicillium marneffei* showing a branched conidiophore and chains of conidia. (Courtesy of Dr D W Warnock, PHLS Mycology Reference Laboratory, Bristol)**

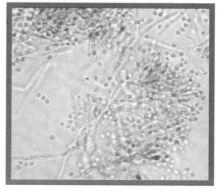

6.2 Opportunistic systemic mycoses

These infections are seen regularly in immunocompromised individuals, including bone marrow transplant recipients, those in intensive care and surgical, neutropenic, cancer and AIDS patients. The underlying condition may determine the clinical presentation of the systemic mycosis, its route and the principal sites of infection and the fungal species involved.

Systemic candidosis

Deep or systemic infections caused by *Candida* species are the commonest of the systemic mycoses in most countries. They are frequently caused by *C. albicans* but an increasing number due to other *Candida* species such as *C. glabrata, C. tropicalis* and *C. krusei* are being encountered. In some hospitals, half the deep *Candida* infections are caused by non-*albicans* species. There are, however, no differences in the clinical manifestations of the infections caused by these different organisms.

Patients are generally infected by the strain of *Candida* which they have been carrying in the body. Occasionally outbreaks of candidosis have been attributed to a common source, as when a particular strain has spread within an intensive care unit (ICU) or neonatal ward. The route of infection, though, may vary. In most neutropenic patients invasion via the gastrointestinal tract is thought to be the main route of entry, whereas in drug abusers it is possible for patients to introduce the organism inadvertently by injection.

Clinical features

The main clinical manifestations are determined by the route of infection and the type of predisposition. For instance, in immunocompetent patients *Candida* infections may localize in the retina and vitreous of the eye where it is more difficult to mount an effector host reaction, whereas in the severely neutropenic patient the infection is often very widespread. However, in many patients the infection may simply present with nonspecific features such as fever, hypotension and malaise. The main clinical features are summarized in **Figure 180**.

It is important to recognize characteristic features of candidosis in certain patients. For instance, hepatosplenic candidosis is difficult to manage and the diagnosis is usually made by the presence of opacities on abdominal CT scans in patients who have neutropenia or have recently recovered from neutropenia and who also have a high pyrexia.

Diarrhea has occasionally been associated with *Candida* but convincing proof that the two are causally related may be lacking even though some patients respond to oral antifungals.

Clinical features of systemic candidosis

Disease	Underlying predisposition	Clinical features
Candida cystitis	Antibiotic therapy, urethral obstruction	Dysuria, frequency, etc.
Deep focal candidosis	Peritoneal dialysis	Pain, distension
	Ureteric obstruction, surgery	Renal pelvis, colic, fever, fungal balls in urine
Candidemia	Many, eg abdominal surgery, cancer	Fever, positive blood culture
Disseminated candidosis	Neutropenia	Fever, muscle pain, skin nodules, papules
	Surgery	Fever, renal failure, metastatic abscesses
	iv heroin abusers	Fever, arthritis, eg costochondral joints, endophthalmitis, severe folliculitis
	Neonatal prematurity	Fever, shock, meningitis, ureteric obstruction
	iv feeding in neonates	Fever, endophthalmitis
	Valve surgery in endocarditis	Fever, large emboli
Hepatosplenic candidosis	Neutropenia (in remission)	High fever, severe malaise, liver enlargement, opacities on CT scan

↑ **Fig. 180**
Clinical features of systemic candidosis.

Laboratory diagnosis

This can be difficult as there is often inadequate laboratory evidence on which to base a diagnosis. Direct microscopy does not play a major role in identifying deep infections although it may be helpful in certain situations such as the detection of hyphal balls in ureteric infections. Cultural isolation of a *Candida* species from a site where it may be a saprophyte, eg the mouth, in a predisposed patient with fever, will need careful interpretation. However, isolation from the blood, cerebrospinal fluid (CSF) or peritoneum is significant and the use of biphasic media or lysis–centrifugation is helpful.

Despite many attempts, there is no ideal system for serologic detection of candidosis either using an antibody or an antigen detection system. Under certain circumstances antibody detection is a valuable procedure, eg in endocarditis or hepatosplenic infection.

Histopathology, if it reveals the presence of yeasts plus hyphae, will confirm the diagnosis (**Fig. 181**).

Management

It is important to identify *Candida* isolates to species level as antifungal sensitivity varies between the different species. *C. glabrata* and *C. krusei* frequently show reduced sensitivity to fluconazole, and *C. lusitaniae* to amphotericin B.

For nonneutropenic patients with *C. albicans* infections fluconazole can be used. For neutropenic patients amphotericin B is usually given. If there is an inadequate response, either a lipid-associated amphotericin B or fluconazole is substituted or flucytosine can be added, provided that renal function is normal. For species such as *C. krusei* and *C. glabrata*, amphotericin B should be given but itraconazole is an alternative.

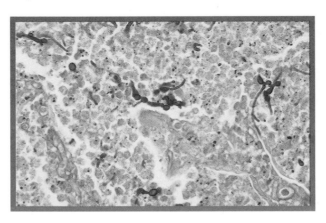

← **Fig. 181 Section of lung showing hyphae and yeasts of *Candida* (PAS stain).**

Aspergillosis

Fungi of the genus *Aspergillus* are well-recognized human pathogens which may cause a variety of conditions depending on the underlying predisposition. The main species involved are *A. fumigatus,* followed by *A. flavus* and *A. niger.* *Aspergillus* species are a common component of the airborne fungal flora and therefore exposure to these fungi is widespread. High environmental loads of spores have been associated with building work, contaminated ventilation systems and compost heaps. The patterns of disease associated with aspergilli are summarized in **Figure 182.**

Colonization

This is common in patients with chronic pulmonary disease such as emphysema or chronic sinusitis. No treatment is required.

Patterns of disease caused by *Aspergillus* species

Colonization
Aspergilloma
        Pulmonary
        Paranasal sinus
Allergic disease
        Asthma, hay fever
        Allergic alveolitis
        Allergic bronchopulmonary aspergillosis
        Allergic *Aspergillus* sinusitis
Invasive aspergillosis
        Acute invasive disease
            Pulmonary
            Paranasal sinus
            Disseminated
        Chronic necrotizing disease
        Paranasal *Aspergillus* granuloma

↑ **Fig. 182**
Patterns of disease caused by *Aspergillus* species.

Aspergilloma

This infection can develop following unrestricted growth of the organisms within a pulmonary cavity or paranasal sinus.

Pulmonary aspergillomas are most often caused by *A. fumigatus*, followed by *A. niger*. Patients usually present with increasing dyspnea and hemoptysis. They generally have an underlying existing lung cavity following tuberculosis, sarcoidosis or other cause such as ankylosing spondylitis. The lesions are found on X-ray or CT scan of the chest and appear as solid lesions within a cavity. This will also be seen in autopsy material (**Fig. 183**). The air crescent sign and movement of the fungal ball can be demonstrated. Microscopy is seldom useful, although expectorated fungal hyphae may provide a clue to the diagnosis (**Fig. 184**). A positive culture of sputum on glucose–peptone agar at 37°C, excluding cycloheximide, will establish the causal organism.

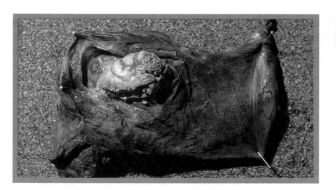

← **Fig. 183
Aspergilloma
in lung.**

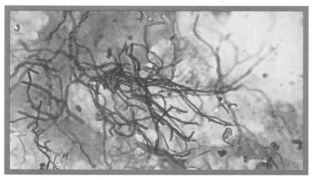

← **Fig. 184
Aspergillus
hyphae in
sputum (Gram
stain).**

Serologic tests are helpful. There are usually very high titers of antibody to *Aspergillus* antigen. For management, surgical removal may be necessary if bleeding occurs. The value of antifungal chemotherapy is not proven.

Aspergillomas of the paranasal sinuses are usually established radiologically in patients with sinus obstruction. They can be removed surgically.

Allergic disease

Inhaled *Aspergillus* spores may give rise to asthma or hay fever. This is managed as with other asthmatic disorders.

Allergic alveolitis with secondary fibrosis has been associated with *A. clavatus*. It occurs in certain occupational groups such as malt workers after inhalation of *Aspergillus* spores and the diagnosis is established serologically. Treatment is with systemic corticosteroids .

Allergic bronchopulmonary aspergillosis (ABPA) may present with reversible dyspnea but later long-term shortness of breath occurs. It is caused by the development of immunologic responses to aspergilli growing within airways. There is peribronchiolar inflammation, and mucous plugs form in the bronchi, leading to segmental atelectasis and bronchial dilatation. A similar condition may affect patients with cystic fibrosis, where aspergilli may contribute to exacerbations of the underlying pathology. The diagnosis of ABPA is established by skin testing and performing both conventional serology and radioallergosorbent tests (RASTs) (for specific IgE) with appropriate *Aspergillus* antigens. Sputum sometimes contains bronchial casts (**Fig. 185**) and sections of

→ Fig. 185
Bronchial casts in sputum.

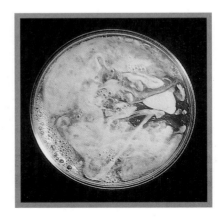

these will show filaments on microscopy (**Fig. 186**). Cultures are often negative.

Allergic *Aspergillus* sinusitis is a similar condition of the paranasal sinuses, which presents with obstruction and a mucoid exudate containing sparse numbers of hyphae and eosinophils. The value of antifungals has not been established in the management of the latter two conditions, and most patients are treated symptomatically with bronchodilators and inhaled or systemic corticosteroids.

Invasive aspergillosis

Acute invasive disease is a life-threatening infection caused by the invasion of the tissues by aspergilli. This infection is usually seen in severely ill patients, particularly those with neutropenia, solid organ transplant recipients, patients with multiorgan failure and those receiving high doses of corticosteroids. AIDS patients may also develop aspergillosis.

The clinical signs of lung invasion are often nonspecific, presenting with fever, cough and pulmonary infiltrates in a predisposed patient. On X-ray a variety of changes from solitary patches of consolidation to pleural effusions may be seen. A characteristic finding is solitary or multiple cavitating lesions with pleural reaction, often best detected by CT scan rather than X-rays, particularly in the early stages of disease. Intrabronchial invasion by aspergilli may also occur, particularly in AIDS patients.

Primary invasion of the paranasal sinuses can occur in severely immunocompromised patients. Facial pain and swelling associated with nasal obstruction and eventually erosion of the palate develop. The extent of infection can be detected by X-ray or CT scan. This pattern of infection is most often associated with *A. flavus*.

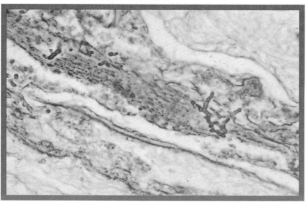

← **Fig. 186 Section of a bronchial cast showing filaments (GMS).**

Infections may disseminate to other sites such as the brain or bone. Rarely, solitary cerebral granulomas can also occur.

The diagnosis of invasive aspergillosis is difficult but can be established by the presence of *Aspergillus* in sputum or bronchoalveolar lavage (BAL) by microscopy and culture. The isolation of *Aspergillus* species from such specimens should be regarded as a potentially sinister sign in neutropenic patients and, if accompanied by appropriate clinical findings, an indication for therapy. Transbronchial biopsies may show invasion of the lung by fungal mycelium and, although not specific for aspergilli, this technique is very helpful (**Fig. 187**). Serology is less helpful in the diagnosis of invasive aspergillosis, although antigen detection is sometimes positive.

In most patients amphotericin B is the treatment of choice. Lipid-associated amphotericin B can also be used when there is little response. A further alternative is itraconazole.

Chronic necrotizing pulmonary aspergillosis is an uncommon condition where there is inflammation with fibrosis, often in patients with a predisposition such as sarcoidosis, chronic corticosteroid therapy or fibrotic lung disease. With progression there is extensive fibrosis and recurrent secondary infections. Weight loss and low-grade fever are common. X-rays show a chronic infiltrate and fibrosis with bronchial dilatation and, occasionally, aspergillomas. Microscopy and culture are seldom consistently positive and tests should be performed repeatedly. Patients usually have raised antibody titers to aspergilli.

Management is with oral itraconazole.

→ Fig. 187 Section of invasive aspergillosis showing dichotomous branching of the hyphae (H&E stain).

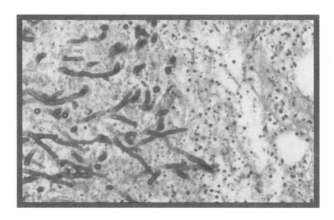

A similar condition, which may occur in the paranasal sinuses, is also treated with itraconazole.

Paranasal *Aspergillus* granuloma is a progressive invasive condition, occurring in nonimmunosuppressed subjects in the tropics; it has a characteristic histopathology with small fragments of hyphae seen within macrophages and giant cells. Its progress is usually relentless. The species involved is *A. flavus*.

Identification of *Aspergillus* species

Colonies of aspergilli develop rapidly on glucose–peptone agar, without cycloheximide, at 37°C.

A. fumigatus has colonies with a smokey green color (**Fig. 188**). The sporing heads seen on microscopy have flask-shaped vesicles which have one row of phialides over the upper two thirds of the surface. The conidia are produced in parallel chains (**Fig. 189**).

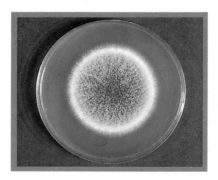

← Fig. 188
Colony of *Aspergillus fumigatus*.

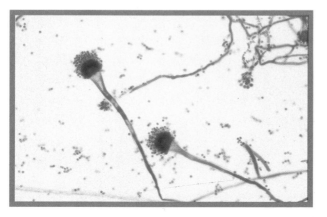

← Fig. 189
Microscopy of *Aspergillus fumigatus* showing flask-shaped vesicles and phialides bearing conidia.

A. flavus colonies are yellow/green in color (**Fig. 190**). The sporing heads have rough-walled conidiophores and globose vesicles which have phialides in one or two rows over the whole surface (**Fig. 191**).

→ Fig. 190
Colony of *Aspergillus flavus*.

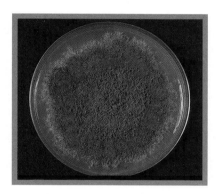

→ Fig. 191
Microscopy of *Aspergillus flavus* showing globose vesicles.

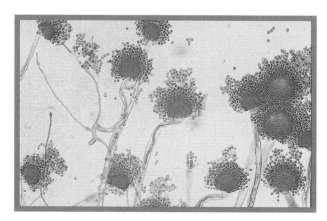

Cryptococcosis

This is an opportunistic fungal infection caused by the encapsulated yeast, *Cryptococcus neoformans*. It has features of an endemic respiratory mycosis although it most frequently occurs in the immunocompromised patient.

There are two variants of the species:
- *C. neoformans* var. *neoformans*, found in nature in pigeon excreta, and
- *C. neoformans* var. *gattii* found in debris from certain species of eucalyptus trees.

Infections occur both in previously healthy individuals, usually in the tropics, and in immunocompromised patients. Underlying predisposing conditions include sarcoidosis, lymphoma, systemic lupus erythematosus (SLE), solid organ transplantation and AIDS, where 3–13% of patients may develop cryptococcal infection. *Cryptococcus* invades the lungs after inhalation and disseminates from this site, causing fungemia and meningitis.

Clinical features

Asymptomatic infection. A few studies have shown a moderate level (15–30%) of skin test positivity in a normal population.

Subacute or chronic pulmonary infection. Patients present with cough, chest pain or fever. X-rays show interstitial infiltrates, hilar lymphadenopathy, miliary nodules, pleural effusion or even widespread uni- or bilateral opacification.

Widely disseminated infections. These are typical of AIDS patients, where positive blood cultures are common.

Infection of the central nervous system (CNS). Headache, neck stiffness, coma and cranial nerve palsy all occur, but these symptoms may be suppressed in AIDS patients.

Skin presentations. These include papules, nodules, ulcers, abscesses and cellulitis.

Other sites. Involvement includes liver, spleen, prostate and bone.

Laboratory diagnosis

Direct microscopy of India ink or Nigrosin preparations of exudates, serum, CSF, etc. will show the yeasts and highlight the capsule (**Fig. 192**).

Culture on glucose–peptone agar without cycloheximide yields yeasts at room temperature but 30°C is preferable. The colonies are shiny and mucoid in texture (**Fig. 193**). Identification of the culture is by biochemical tests.

On serology, antigen can be demonstrated in serum or CSF using latex agglutination or an enzyme-linked immunosorbent assay (ELISA) method. False-positive latex tests may be seen in patients with circulating antiglobulins, such as rheumatoid factors, which can be removed by heating. Antibody levels are not helpful for diagnosis.

→ Fig. 192
India ink
preparation of
CSF showing
the yeasts of
*Cryptococcus
neoformans*
surrounded by
a wide
capsule.

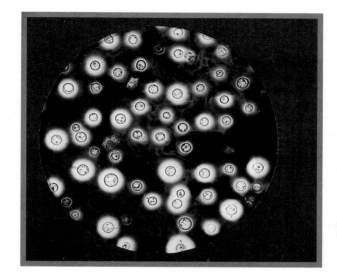

→ Fig. 193
Colony of
*Cryptococcus
neoformans.*

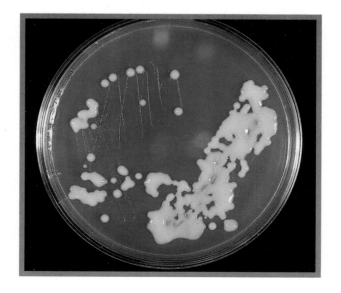

Histopathology of sections shows large yeasts (8–15µm) with capsules of variable sizes. The capsular material will stain with a mucicarmine stain (**Fig. 194**). Occasionally, small yeasts, which resemble *Candida* species, are seen.

Features of cryptococcosis in AIDS patients include:
- a high frequency of positive blood cultures,
- high antigen titers in serum which are often greater than those in CSF
- the slow fall of antigen levels with therapy.

Management

For nonAIDS patients amphotericin B and flucytosine are usually given for a minimum of 4 weeks, longer in the immunocompromised patient. For AIDS patients amphotericin B, with or without flucytosine, is used for 2 weeks followed by fluconazole. An alternative for long-term suppression is itraconazole.

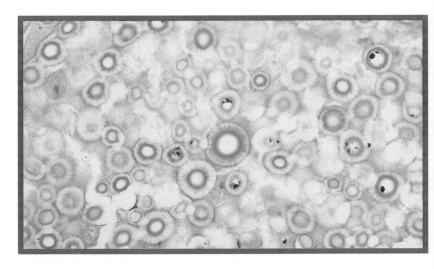

↑ **Fig. 194**
Section showing capsulated yeasts (mucicarmine).

Zygomycosis

This is an opportunistic infection caused by fungi of the genera *Rhizomucor, Rhizopus* and *Absidia*. These zygomycete fungi produce large, strap-shaped hyphae with no, or few, septa. They are environmental saprophytes and include the common pin molds found on stale food. Rarer causes include species of *Cunninghamella* and *Saksenaea*.

Infections caused by these fungi are rare. Outbreaks due to certain *Rhizopus* species have been associated with exposure to specific hazards such as contaminated dressing packs. The different types of infection and the associated predisposing factors are given in **Figure 195**.

Clinical features

All zygomycosis cases are associated with tissue infarction caused by infiltration of blood vessels and subsequent necrosis. The commonest form, rhinocerebral zygomycosis, presents with edema and erythema over the cheek with progressive periorbital swelling and visual impairment. It is most often seen in poorly controlled diabetics, although a slower variant is seen rarely in those with milder diabetes.

Cutaneous zygomycosis presents with necrosis and infarction around a burn or compound fracture site with a rapidly extending margin of edema. Pulmonary mucormycosis does not have typical features but is usually diagnosed in the neutropenic patient under investigation for respiratory disease.

Zygomycosis and underlying predisposition

Clinical pattern of infection	Predisposing factor
Rhinocerebral	Diabetes mellitus
Pulmonary, disseminated	Neutropenia
Cutaneous	Burns
Gastrointestinal	Malnutrition

↑ **Fig. 195**
Zygomycosis and underlying predisposition.

Laboratory diagnosis

Direct microscopy of aspirates, sputum, etc. may show the diagnostic broad strap-like hyphae. Impression smears of cut tissue or even frozen sections have been used for rapid detection. Histopathology, which shows wide hyphae branching at right angles is diagnostic (**Fig. 196**). Cultures on glucose–peptone agar, excluding cycloheximide, will yield molds that have a fibrous texture and rapidly fill the Petri dish. However, cultures of material with microscopically proven infection may fail to grow. Species such as *Absidia corymbifera* and *Rhisopus arrhizus* are causes of this infection (**Figs 197–199**).

No serologic tests are available.

Management

Usually amphotericin B, either normal or in a lipid-associated formulation is used.

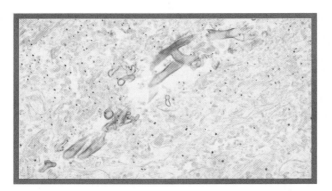

← Fig. 196 Section of zygomycosis showing wide hyphae with perpendicular branching (PAS).

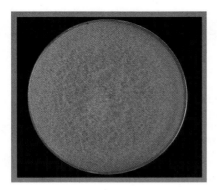

← Fig. 197 Colony of *Absidia corymbifera*.

→ **Fig. 198**
Microscopy of
Absidia
corymbifera.
The sporangia
have a funnel-
shaped base
and a
pronounced
columella.

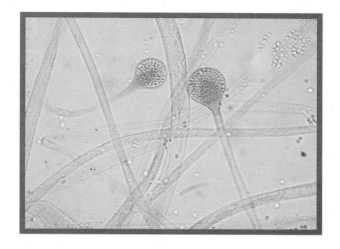

→ **Fig. 199**
Microscopy of
Rhizopus
arrhizus
showing
sporangio-
phores arising
from rhizoids.
The sporangia
are large and
collapse at
maturity,
leaving the
wall attached
to the
sporangio-
phore.

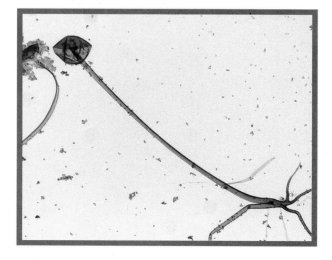

Other opportunistic mycoses

It is inevitable that, where patients have little or no resistance to infection, unusual organisms may cause disease. This is certainly true of the fungi, and from time to time unusual pathogens can be identified in severely ill patients. The best recognized of these are *Trichosporon, Fusarium* and *Acremonium* species, *Scedosporium apiospermum* and *S. inflatum*. These organisms have few characteristics which allow the clinician to identify them without culture.

If an unusual organism is identified in an immunocompromised patient it should be regarded as a potential pathogen although it is important to consider whether it is merely colonizing an appropriate site.

Management

The broadest-spectrum antifungal is amphotericin B, which should be used, although *S. apiospermum* may respond to intravenous miconazole.

7 | Antifungal Agents

The modern antifungals comprise three main families of drugs and a large number of additional compounds which make up a miscellaneous group of agents.

The first of the major antifungal families was the polyene group which contains compounds all derived from *Streptomyces* species. The main drugs in use today are:
- amphotericin B, including lipid-associated formulations,
- nystatin
- natamycin.

The large azole family now has two subgroups, the imidazoles and the triazoles. They are all synthetic drugs with a common mode of action. Examples are given in **Figure 200**. The third group, the allylamines – terbinafine and naftifine – are also synthetic drugs.

Subgroups of the azole antifungal agents

Imidazoles	Triazoles
Miconazole	Itraconazole
Econazole	Fluconazole
Ketoconazole	etc.
Clotrimazole	
Tioconazole	
etc.	

↑ **Fig. 200**
Subgroups of the azole antifungal agents.

There is also a large miscellaneous group of antifungals. Those used most frequently are:

- griseofulvin,
- flucytosine,
- amorolfine,
- tolnaftate and
- cyclopiroxolamine.

The modes of action of these drugs vary (**Fig. 201**). The majority affect the integrity of the cell membrane. Antifungals which block other processes include flucytosine, which affects RNA and DNA synthesis. Most antifungal drugs in laboratory tests inhibit the growth of fungi (fungistatic) at the concentrations achievable at the sites of infection but a few are able to destroy the organisms (fungicidal). The difference may be important clinically where host resistance is impaired or otherwise ineffective. The use of antifungals is shown in **Figure 202**.

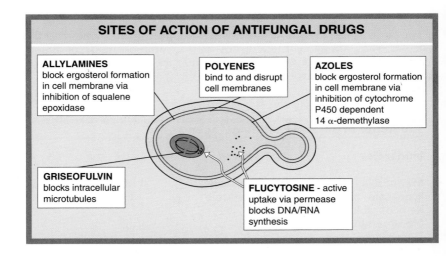

SITES OF ACTION OF ANTIFUNGAL DRUGS

ALLYLAMINES
block ergosterol formation in cell membrane via inhibition of squalene epoxidase

POLYENES
bind to and disrupt cell membranes

AZOLES
block ergosterol formation in cell membrane via inhibition of cytochrome P450 dependent 14 α-demethylase

GRISEOFULVIN
blocks intracellular microtubules

FLUCYTOSINE - active uptake via permease blocks DNA/RNA synthesis

↑ **Fig. 201**
Sites of action of antifungal drugs.

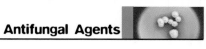

The use of antifungal drugs

Drugs	Fungi affected	Formulation
Amphotericin B	*Candida*, systemic	Topical, iv
Nystatin	*Candida*	Topical
Natamycin	*Candida*, dermatophytes	Topical
Miconazole	Superficial Some systemic not *Aspergillus*	Topical, iv
Clotrimazole	Superficial	Topical
Econazole	Superficial	Topical
Tioconazole	Superficial	Topical
Ketoconazole	Superficial Some systemic not *Aspergillus*	Topical, oral
Itraconazole	Superficial, systemic	Oral
Fluconazole	Superficial Systemic not *Aspergillus*	Oral, iv
Terbinafine	Dermatophytes Some deep, e.g. Sporotrichosis Chromoblastomycosis	Topical, oral
Griseofulvin	Dermatophytes	Oral
Flucytosine	*Candida*, *Cryptococcus*	Oral, iv
Amorolfine	Superficial	Topical
Tolnaftate	Dermatophytes	Topical
Cyclopiroxolamine	Superficial	Topical

↑ **Fig. 202**
The use of antifungal drugs.

Further reading

Campbell CK, Johnson EM, Philpot CM, Warnock DW. Identification of pathogenic fungi. London: Public Health Laboratory Service, 1996.

Chandler FW, Watts JC. Pathologic diagnosis of fungal infections. Chicago: ASCP, 1987.

deHoog GS, Guarro J, eds. Atlas of clinical fungi. Baarn: Centraalbureau voor Schimmelcultures, 1996.

Elewski BE, ed. Cutaneous fungal infections. New York: Igaku-Shoin, 1992.

Evans EGV, Richardson MD, eds. Medical mycology: a practical approach. Oxford: IRL Press, 1989.

Hawksworth DL, Kirk PM, Sutton BC, Pegler DN. Dictionary of the fungi. Wallingford: CAB International, 1995.

Kibbler CC, Mackenzie DWR, Odds FC. Principles and practice of clinical mycology. Chichester: Wiley, 1996.

Koneman EW, Roberts GD. Practical laboratory mycology, 3E. Baltimore: Williams and Wilkins, 1985.

Kwon-Chung KJ, Bennett JE. Medical mycology. Philadelphia: Lea & Febiger, 1992.

Odds FC. Candida and candidosis, 2E. London: Baillière Tindall, 1988.

Richardson MD, Warnock DW. Fungal infection, diagnosis and management. Oxford: Blackwell Scientific, 1993.

Rippon JW. Medical mycology. The pathogenic fungi and the pathogenic actinomycetes, 3E. Philadelphia: WB Saunders, 1988.

Salfelder K. Atlas of fungal pathology. Dordrecht: Kluwer, 1990.

Samaranayake LP, MacFarlane TW, eds. Oral candidosis, 2E. London: Wright, 1990.

St-Germain G, Summerbell R. Identifying filamentous fungi. Belmont, USA: Star, 1996.

Warnock DW, Richardson MD, eds. Fungal infection in the compromised patient, 2E. Chichester: Wiley, 1991.

INDEX

Page numbers in **bold** refer to figures

A

Absidia corymbifera, 144, **145**
Absidia spp. 117, 143
acne **74**
Acremonium, spp.
  nail infection, 84
  severely ill patients, 146
Acremonium strictum, 84–5
Actinomadura madurae, **97**, **101**
Actinomadura pellietieri, **97**, **98**
actinomycetes, mycetoma, 97, 101
actinomycetoma, 95, 101
AIDS
  aspergillosis, 136
  candidosis, 7
    chronic pseudomembranous, 60
    esophageal 61
    oral 59
  cryptococcosis, 117, 140, 142
  dermatophytosis, 7–8
  histoplasmosis, 119
  Penicillium marneffei infection, 128, 129
  seborrheic dermatitis, 75
  subungual onychomycosis, 25
allergic alveolitis, 135
allergic bronchopulmonary aspergillosis, 135
allergic response, 6
allylamines, 147
alopecia areata, 42
Alternaria alternata, 110
amikacin, 101
amorolfine, 57, 71, 85, 148, **149**
amphoterocin B, 71, 101, 109, 147, **149**
  candidosis, 132
  coccidiomycosis, 122
  cryptococcosis, 142
  histoplasmosis, 121
  invasive aspergillosis, 137
  opportunistic mycoses, 146
  Penicillium marneffei infection, 129
  zygomycosis, 144
angular cheilitis, 61
antifungal agents, 147–8, **149**
  sites of action, **148**
  use, **149**
  see also individual agents
arthroconidia, 7, 12
Ascomycota, 1
ascospores, 1
aspergilloma 134–5

aspergillosis, 5, 117, 133–9
  allergic disease, 135–6
  bronchial casts in sputum, 135–6
  chronic necrotizing pulmonary, 137
  disease patterns **133**
  invasive 136–8
Aspergillus antigen 135
Aspergillus clavatus 135
Aspergillus flavus 133, 136, 139
Aspergillus fumigatus, 92, 133, 134, 138
Aspergillus niger, 90, **91**, 133, 134
Aspergillus spp., 117
  culture temperature, 14
  identification, 138–9
  nail infection, 84
asteroid body, 103
asthma, 6
azaleic acid, 72
azoles, 71
  seborrheic dermatitis treatment, 76

B

Basidiobolus haptosporus, 112, **113**, 114
Basidiobolus ranarum, **115**
Basidiomycota, 1
basidiospores, 1
Behçet's syndrome, 62
benzoic acid, 57
betadine, 71
Bipolaris spp., 111
Blastomyces dermatitidis, 117, 124, **125**
blastomycosis, 117, 124–6
brush culture, 10, **11**

C

Candida albicans, 7, 8, 58
  chlamydospores, **70**
  culture, **69**
  with diaper dermatitis, 63
  germ tubes, **70**
  nail infection, 64
  systemic infection, 130, 132
  vaginal infection, 62
Candida glabrata, 58, 130, 132
  vaginal infection, 62
Candida granuloma, 66
Candida intertrigo, 63
Candida krusei, 58, 130, 132
Candida lusitaniae, 132
Candida parapsilosis, 58
  nail infection, 64, **65**
Candida spp., 5
  culture temperature, 14

keratitis, 92
onychomycosis differential diagnosis, **25**
opportunist, 117
otomycosis 90
Candida tropicalis, 58, 130
  vaginal infection, 62
candidemia, **131**
candidosis
  angular cheilitis, 61
  chronic mucocutaneous, 61, 65, 66–7, 71
  chronic nodular, 61
  chronic plaque-like, 60, 61
  cystitis, **131**
  deep focal, **131**
  disseminated, **131**
  erythematous, 60, 61
  esophageal, 61
  groin, 26, 63
  hepatosplenic, 130, **131**
  infection factors, **8**
  oropharyngeal, 7
  predisposing factors, 58
  pseudomembranous
    acute, 59
    chronic, 60
candidosis, superficial, 58–71
  clinical features, 58
  cutaneous, 66
  diaper dermatitis, 63
  endogenous, 58
  interdigital, 64
  laboratory diagnosis, 68, **69–70**
  management, 71
  nails, 64–5
  oral, 58, 59–61
  pathology, 58
  vaginal, 58, 62, 66, 71
candidosis, systemic, 117, 130, **131**, 132
  clinical features, 130, **131**
  diagnosis, 132
  infection route, 130
  management, 132
cerebral granuloma, aspergillosis, 137
chlamydospores
  Candida albicans, **70**
  Trichophyton tonsurans, 46
chromoblastomycosis, 95, 106–9
  diagnosis, 107–8
  management, 109
Cladosporium carrionii, 8, 108
clotrimazole, 71, **147**, **149**
co-trimoxazole, 101
Coccidioides immitis, 117, 122, **123**
coccidioidomycosis, 117, 122, **123**